"As the relationship between our body and creative imagination moves increasingly to center stage in the research of our human condition – in studies of trauma, creativity, psychotherapy, placebo, biology, artificial intelligence and the arts – along comes a book that pulls it all together. With scholarly accuracy and solid research into a wide variety of fields that underlie theory formation in the study of psychotherapy as a creative art, Dr Leanne Domash has written a book I had been waiting for. While eminently practical and full of case examples, it shows scientific undercurrents in the rapidly changing science of psychotherapy and creativity. Their foundations in neuroscience, biology and chaos theory are explained in an elegant and fully embodied style we can all understand."

Robert Bosnak, PsyA, Jungian psychoanalyst, originator of the Embodied Imagination method; Teaching Instructor at SUNY Upstate Medical University, Department of Psychiatry.

"If I had chosen another life path as a religious leader, I would bless this book for tackling the role of uncertainty and faith within psychotherapy. And there is so much more to be had. Author Leanne Domash covers many thorny topics at the heart of healing—the role of desire, inspiration, surprise, strangeness, intuition, and wonder. This is a Wonderland of a book, a dream space, an alchemical kettle for simmering creativity and imagination. By revealing her own doubts and vulnerabilities along the way, Domash walks her talk while providing a unique and persuasive synthesis of research that points towards an inherently creative universe, right down to the cellular level. This is a must read for all therapists wishing to enhance their creative faculties."

Terry Marks-Tarlow, PhD, clinical psychologist, Santa Monica, CA; author of *Psyche's Veil*, *Clinical Intuition in Psychotherapy* and *A Fractal Epistemology for a Scientific Psychology*

"Drawing upon thousands of years of insights into the vast potential of human imagination from the Kabbalists and Maimonides to current psychoanalytic theory and neuropsychology, Leanne Domash offers us not simply a book to read but a space in which to explore and expand our notions of psychotherapeutic healing, the use of dreams, the vast potential locked in the therapeutic relationship and the emergence of the therapist's own unique voice. This profoundly rich book compellingly opens up a unique perspective on the many ways that imagination and creativity are at the core of psychotherapeutic healing and authentic living itself."

Robert Grossmark, PhD, ABPP, NYU Postdoctoral Program in Psychoanalysis and Psychotherapy; author of *The Unobtrusive Relational Analyst: Explorations in Psychoanalytic Companioning*

Imagination, Creativity and Spirituality in Psychotherapy

The aim of this book is to awaken creative desire and expand the imagination of the psychotherapist and, in turn, her patient. Each chapter is meant to surprise the reader and help him see the world in a new way. Many varieties of imagination are explored – the spiritual, the relational, the dreamworld, the aesthetic and the adaptive. The author offers space to reflect, to daydream, to remember; space to pursue goals, to make new connections; space to take risks and space to be wrong. The psychotherapist is encouraged to find her own voice, be poetic, dare to create, converse with other disciplines and, most especially, enter the world of dreams. This is all passed onto the patient as the dyad enters the intersubjective field.

Both scholarly and practical, this volume elegantly and persuasively synthesizes *for the first time* research in many fields, including spirituality and Kabbalah, neuroscience, the arts, biology and artificial intelligence, to give an in depth and original understanding of the current pressing problems in the rapidly changing field of psychotherapy: how do we work with unconscious processes and early memories to help our patients become more imaginative, creative, hopeful and resilient, and in so doing, heal. The relationship between the body and creative imagination is fully explored as well as the disruptive effect of trauma on the imagination and how to address this.

The emphasis on surprise, uncanny communication, interdisciplinary inquiry, use of dreamwork and the imagination of the body — how it spontaneously meets new challenges — all stimulate the creativity of the reader. Through numerous case studies, the author illustrates the practical implications of how this exploration allows for deeper understanding and more effective treatment. With the innovative synthesis and specific techniques the author provides, the clinician has tools to carry on the work of moving the field of psychotherapy forward as well as work ever more effectively with patients.

Dr. Leanne Domash has had a life-long interest in the creative process and the intersection of imagination, spirituality and psychotherapy. She is a psychologist/psychoanalyst, writer and playwright and Certified Embodied Imagination Practitioner. Dr. Domash has written and spoken widely about the creative process, the uses of imagination, the healing power of art, the value of dreamwork and the implicit spirituality embedded in the psychotherapy process.

Dr. Domash is Clinical Consultant in the New York University Postdoctoral Program in Psychotherapy and Psychoanalysis; Voluntary Psychologist, Mt. Sinai Beth Israel Medical Center, New York, NY; Associate Clinical Professor of Psychiatry, Icahn School of Medicine at Mt. Sinai, New York, NY. She maintains a private practice in New York.

Psyche and Soul

The *Psyche and Soul: Psychoanalysis, Spirituality and Religion in Dialogue* series explores the intersection of psychoanalysis, spirituality and religion. By promoting dialogue, this series provides a platform for the vast and expanding interconnections, mutual influences and points of divergence amongst these disciplines. Extending beyond western religions of Judaism, Christianity and Islam, the series includes Eastern religions, contemplative studies, mysticism and philosophy. By bridging gaps, opening the vistas and responding to increasing societal yearnings for more spirituality in psychoanalysis, *Psyche and Soul* aims to cross these disciplines, fostering a more fluid interpenetration of ideas.

For a full list of titles in this series, please visit the Routledge website: https://www.routledge.com/Psyche-and-Soul/book-series/PSYSOUL

Imagination, Creativity and Spirituality in Psychotherapy

Welcome to Wonderland

Leanne Domash, PhD

Routledge
Taylor & Francis Group
LONDON AND NEW YORK

First published 2021
by Routledge
2 Park Square, Milton Park, Abingdon, Oxon OX14 4RN

and by Routledge
52 Vanderbilt Avenue, New York, NY 10017

Routledge is an imprint of the Taylor & Francis Group, an informa business

British Library Cataloguing-in-Publication Data
A catalogue record for this book is available from the British Library

Library of Congress Cataloging-in-Publication Data
Names: Domash, Leanne, author.
Title: The role of imagination, creativity and spirituality in psychotherapy: welcome to wonderland / Leanne Domash, PhD.
Identifiers: LCCN 2020013878 | ISBN 9780367280024 (hardback) | ISBN 9780367280031 (paperback) | ISBN 9780429299148 (ebook)
Subjects: LCSH: Imagination—Therapeutic use. | Creation (Literary, artistic, etc.)—Therapeutic use. | Psychotherapy.
Classification: LCC RC489.F35 D66 2020 | DDC 616.89/14—dc23
LC record available at https://lccn.loc.gov/2020013878

ISBN: 978-0-367-28002-4 (hbk)
ISBN: 978-0-367-28003-1 (pbk)
ISBN: 978-0-429-29914-8 (ebk)

Typeset in Times New Roman
by codeMantra

Dedicated to my husband Kenneth Theil
for his vast love, gentle support
and uncanny ability to make me laugh

Contents

Acknowledgments

I wish to thank so many people and objects for help in writing this book. Let me start with my undergraduate education at the University of Chicago. I thank Mr. Rosenheim who took our Humanities Class to Orchestra Hall to hear T.S. Eliot read *The Love Song of J. Alfred Prufrock*; the long-forgotten-named professor who taught me about the prophets of the Old Testament; the worn-out leather chair in the Poetry Library where I sat and read for hours; and the kindly matron who provided clean sheets and a wake-up call in the anteroom of the Ladies Room of Cobb Hall so students could power nap on comfortable cots between classes. Oh, and don't let me forget, the generous patron who donated his/her modern art collection so undergraduates (and *only* undergraduates) could hang masterpieces on their dorm room walls. Thanks to this, I had a revolving series of original Klees, Picassos and Mondrians to ponder. Last in this list is the Robie House, designed by Frank Lloyd Wright, that I overlooked from my dorm window.

Fast forward to almost today and I thank Robbie Bosnak and Jill Fischer and the LA3 Class for my practice of Embodied Imagination, a post-Jungian form of dreamwork developed by Robbie that facilitates the imagination. I studied with this group intensively for three years and received a Certificate as an Embodied Imagination Practitioner. I am happy our LA3 class is continuing to study together. As a result of this course, I am able to help patients expand their imagination and also fulfill a lifelong personal ambition to create and produce a number of theatrical presentations. I especially want to thank my director, Jarred Sharar, who has been beside me throughout, for his inspiration, professionalism and good humor.

On a very personal note, I thank my loving, spiritual husband Ken Theil, who provided the facilitating environment for the creation of this book. I am also grateful to my thoughtful, imaginative and adventurous children, Daniel Shapiro and Rachel Shapiro, and their loving partners, Cari Fais and Tom Goren. They all regularly inspire as well as keep me honest lest I drown in overwork. My grandchildren, Penn Shapiro, Isabel Shapiro, Josephine Shapiro and Phoenix Goren, are all beacons helping me envision and embrace the future. To my sister Nanette Goldstein for her support and finally, to my late dear brother Jack; his tenderness, wit and humor will always be remembered.

And to my loving friends and colleagues: Efrat Ginot and Prem Ramchandani for their love, steadfast support and delicious meals and to Wilma and Esteban Cordero, Leslie and Harvey Weinberg, Linda Gunsberg, Terry Marks-Tarlow, David Roane, Judy Marlow, Sam Sanberg, Joel Mitnick, Nina Cerfolio, Randall Shown and Marcos Moscoso for their remarkable inspiration and constant encouragement. I am especially grateful to Efrat Ginot whose perceptive questioning helped me clarify many points. Terry Marks-Tarlow has been very generous in imparting her expertise about the relatively new science of fractals as well as the development of the implicit realm. Ken Theil, Rachel Shapiro and Tom Goren read parts of the manuscript and made excellent suggestions. I thank Ariyele Ressler for her friendship and for offering a gateway to understanding neuroplasticity, including by example. I am very grateful to designer Randall Shown and contractor Marcos Moscoso for creating the sacred space in which to write this book. To my fellow dreamers as we continue our work in Embodied Imagination – Narandja Eagelson, Per (Pelle) Nordin, Kevin Connerton, Meg Kane, Ingrid Blidberg and Rebecca Peterson – for their depth and caring and skill. To colleagues Michael Vannoy Adams for his astute exploration of imagination and Michael Eigen for his many poetic writings on psychoanalysis and spirituality. To my cousin and friend Rhonda Lehr, who tragically died before her time, for being so loving and making me laugh. I still cry for you. To my very talented comrades in theater: illustrious director and actor Jarred Sharar, videographer Ryan Gates and actors Tammy Kopko, Cindy Pearlman, Lisa Gail, Jessica Asch, Russ Roten and Jason Conover for giving my words life. To my empathic and brilliant physician, Dr. Ian Lustbader, who always has a remedy for whatever ails you. To my editor, Carole Maso, for her kind yet authoritative guidance. I love you all.

And, finally, to Jill Salberg, Melanie Suchet and Marie Hoffman, editors of the *Psyche and Soul* book series, for their astute suggestions and faith, support and belief in me.

Chapter 1

Arrival in Wonderland

I am eight or nine years old, sitting in my living room, reading and rereading *Alice's Adventures in Wonderland.* I am entranced by the changing sizes and shapes, the absurd characters, the courage of Alice and the dreamy music of the writing. *Alice* proves a wonderful antidote to the overall conservatism of the small Pennsylvanian town in which I live and to my family's practice of Orthodox Judaism, especially my literal understanding of the multiple rules I thought I had to follow.

I attended an orthodox Hebrew School beginning at age six. The class consisted mostly of boys, and they behaved like the Red Queen but on steroids. The boys were frequently yelling and screaming, racing around the room as well as running out of the room, while the dignified, modest Rabbi ran after them. I sat quietly (perhaps absurdly so, in retrospect) with hands folded, absorbing each and every dictum the Rabbi told us, whenever he had a chance to teach. When I asked my equally modest and scholarly father what I should do about the behavior in class, his only advice was to be "tolerant." Shortly afterward, my secular teacher in school wrote on my report card that she was worried that I was too "serious" in school, meaning I was very rule observant and not playful. Pleased at my restraint, my father wrote back how happy he was to receive the news!

Alice helped me with this state of repression. She, like I, felt confused and bewildered. Yet she learned to challenge authority figures and find her own voice, and she passed some of her newfound knowledge onto me. I, too, gradually found my voice, including challenging my father. Essentially, Alice showed me how "make-believe" can help us see the world from a whole new point of view.

In his wildly imaginative way, Lewis Carroll drew me down into the unconscious, a dreamworld where reorganization and change can occur. I view my childhood reading of *Wonderland* as an interaction of unconscious imaginative processes between Alice and myself, just as Lawrence Zelnick (2014) writes about his reading of Biblical texts, how the readings are imaginative and interpersonal. Alice had begun to think "that very few things indeed were really impossible" (Carroll, 2015, p. 10), and I believed her that something interesting was bound to happen. I continued on from there, and while I took a more academic route than imaginative, I knew my creativity was somewhere inside. In these ways, Alice was my first psychoanalyst.

Another of my "psychoanalysts" is the Jungian analyst Robert Bosnak, creator of the dreamwork technique Embodied Imagination (EI). I heard him speak and sensed this technique, which facilitates the dreamer embodying the images in his dream, would help me expand creatively. I subsequently completed an intensive three-year training course with Bosnak to be an EI practitioner. Along the way, I participated in many experiences using EI, including two brief, in-depth therapies[1] using this technique. As a result, my imagination has expanded, and I have written plays, poems and academic articles. Similar to reading *Wonderland*, learning EI gave me space to imagine. Though still difficult and often a struggle, I have been achieving my goals.

To clarify my therapeutic point of view, I will be using the designation therapist/psychotherapist to mean psychodynamic psychotherapist, as I intend an overall psychodynamic or, in a very broad sense, psychoanalytic orientation. By this I mean a focus on unconscious processes, awareness of implicit meanings, use of dreamwork when applicable and emotionally understanding the origin of unconscious repetitive dysfunctional patterns and how to change them. Many of the references are from the psychoanalytic literature, and when I discuss these sources, I use the term "analyst" or "psychoanalyst," as that is their reference point. However, for our purposes, these terms also refer to therapist/psychotherapist, as similar principles apply. Further, I expand the traditional meaning of psychodynamic psychotherapy to include acknowledgement of the value and importance of imagination, creativity and spirituality in psychotherapy. These factors, in particular, help the patient find hope and meaning and, if relevant, work through trauma. The healing power of the arts is emphasized.

The anxiety of creation

There has been anxiety about writing this book. Anxiety, in fact, may be a necessary component of creation. I struggled with doubt, fearful if I used my authentic voice, I would sound naïve, perhaps ridiculous, and if I chose my academic voice, I would be boring and uninteresting. Although I am a fairly even-tempered person, my experience of writing this book has been kind of "bi-polar-y." There were days when I felt high and very confident about the ideas and the writing. Other days I felt the opposite – depressed, feeling that maybe I just can't do it. With the help of Jill Salberg, one of my editors in the *Psyche and Soul* book series, I found Carole Maso, expert teacher and fiction writer, who gave me courage to experiment, try and re-try, write and rewrite, until my voice began to take shape.

Before I contacted her, the book (which I had already been writing for six months) seemed like a mass of deadened chaos, like a patient who feels scattered and insecure, has flashes of insight but no cohesion, no consistent voice. I needed a mentor, like a patient needs a therapist – an adept presence, a container – to help me properly "form" my creation, or perhaps more accurately, to let my creation become what it wants to be.

Let's look at it this way. Pretend a woman has just had a child. The child has inborn capabilities, but it takes time for various processes to "come online." The child may feel very scattered internally and unable to self-regulate. He or she needs the interaction with the mother/caretaker to feel unified. The caretaker doesn't reject parts of the infant but rather, empathically and authoritatively, tries to help the child integrate these parts. Most importantly, the caretaker helps the child become whom he or she is meant to be. The child's self emerges out of this transitional space between caretaker and child.

This is a relational notion of development, which I translate to both psychotherapy and creativity. Relative chaos is an inherent part of the process in both human development and creativity. Yet, while it is important to tolerate chaos and formlessness, we can't stay in this state too long or we drift into despair. The mentor helps guide us out. For example, a psychotherapist's initial meetings with a patient may feel formless. He or she may have many feelings/thoughts about the patient that are not organized, that don't even make sense. The patient, too, may feel bewildered. Form starts to take shape slowly as both therapist and patient cocreate a meaningful narrative and slowly integrate various self-states.

Just as clinicians serve as mentors to their patients, I hope I will serve as a mentor to you, my reader. This relational aspect of imagination and creativity is a powerfully interesting and necessary ingredient in the process, although the extent of the relational aspect will vary from person to person and project to project. Psychoanalyst and highly influential writer Donald Winnicott definitely subscribed to the relational model of creativity. The transformative effect that his wife and collaborator Clare had on his creativity and productivity has been well documented (Kahr, 1996; Rodman, 2003; Kanter, 2004a,b). Joel Kanter (2004b, p. 457) gives an example by quoting a 1946 letter Donald poignantly wrote to Clare:

> my work is really quite a lot associated with you. Your effect on me is to make me keen and productive and this is all the more awful – because when I am cut off from you I feel paralyzed for all action and originality.

Winnicott saw his creativity as emerging out of the matrix of their relationship.

Hopes and goals

Inspired by Alice, I have several goals in writing this book. First, I aim to help the clinician find her creative voice. This includes claiming one's own synthesis of theories and techniques in the field and letting this synthesis evolve. It also encompasses the clinician's use of language, choosing words that are concise, elegant and lovingly jolting. Language carries with it the essence of the therapeutic relationship. Clinicians are not poets but can aspire to their power.

This will facilitate helping the patient find his or her genuine and most developed sense of self. I am not just referring to the "real" as opposed to the "false" self. By genuine and developed, I mean a refined true self that has verve, tact and novel ways of approaching the world. To paraphrase Alexis de Tocqueville, this is the real self rightly understood.[2]

I also hope to provide the clinician with tools to imagine her own projects into being: giving that presentation, tackling that paper, starting that book. With this in mind, I will catalog some of my anxieties as I write this book. I strive for a balance between reveal and conceal so the reader has enough information to sense my journey with the hope that this will move him toward actualizing his own vision with flair and resourcefulness. However, even with support, the struggle of the creative process is daunting and full of uncertainty and doubt. Even the best parent or therapist cannot (and should not) save his child or patient from trials and anxieties.

I have found the best antidote to doubt is to find faith and hope, that is, to enter transitional space so there is a free flow of ideas and sense of imaginative possibility, and, finally, to give oneself time. It takes so much time to let ideas/feelings/images percolate and then understand how these may be interconnected. Aspiring creators must be realistic about this factor and be willing to give projects generous amounts of time and devotion.

Bosnak (2018) speaks about inviting creative genius into one's life. He stresses that one is "struck" by genius. Genius does not come from the individual but from the material. The individual works with this spark but is careful not to impose on the project or patient. This is especially interesting because it encourages listening to the "material" instead of trying to be in charge of creating. My anxiety, especially at the beginning of writing this book, was because I thought I had to be in charge. I didn't realize the material would work with me and give me direction and guidance.

Second, I hope to awaken and expand creative desire so the clinician can do the same for her patient. Agency and creativity are fueled by desire. Patients need the driving force of desire to enliven their ability to tackle issues and gain momentum to achieve goals. They must want – and want intensely – to undertake the work of psychotherapy. Creative desire is to be distinguished from narcissistic desire, which can interfere with creativity and end in futility. Narcissistic desire is the craving for admiration and validation, frequently accompanied by grandiosity, which can be paralyzing. There can be such a strong need to be validated that the relationship to the work is lost.

Like the patient, the clinician also feels creative desire: to work with unconscious processes to make the implicit explicit, to help the patient identify and rework dysfunctional patterns and have the patient find his authentic self. Clinicians also desire that the patient know them. This leads to interesting countertransference experiences. Which patients have a good sense of the therapist? Which patients appear to have very little? One woman told me recently, "We have no relationship," and pointed to the monetary exchange for services as proof. As she said this, I felt as if I were being punched by something very cold. She had no conscious desire to know me. Can I or should I create a warmth of desire? I did appeal to her wish to have better relationships by explaining how exploring and developing our relationship might facilitate this. However, her deep wounds, still largely secreted away, remain largely out of range of our work. Yet I maintain hope for her and can imagine her learning to tolerate and navigate desire.

While clinicians do have desires, they are also mindful of psychoanalyst Wilfred Bion's exhortation, to enter each session without memory or desire. Therapists must be open to unexpected developments. In this sense, therapists are (metaphorically) like the potter in the book of Jeremiah. At first the potter seems to be controlling what he makes, what it will look like, whether it will be discarded or kept, and so on. But then, according to the very imaginative biblical scholar Avivah Zornberg (1995), the object starts to decide. The potter (therapist) does not have control. He has to work with the object and eventually *the object tells its creator what it will be.* Therapists need the imagination to foresee the future for the patient yet also the imagination to be surprised and let the patient tell us herself.

A third goal is to encourage clinicians to explore the varieties of imagination open to them and their patients: the spiritual, the relational, the dreamworld, the aesthetic and the adaptive. Each provides a basis for creative living. Arnold Modell (2008) writes that we are meant to express what is unique about ourselves, to self-actualize. This begins with freedom of the imagination, which leads to agency and the creation of new meanings. Modell refers to imagination as open, flexible consciousness, which can become constricted by trauma.

I will discuss how to cultivate various types of imagination. Although these will be explored separately, in reality they overlap and intertwine. *Spiritual imagination*, Chapter 2, helps the dyad enter the transitional realm, an implicitly spiritual space. This is crucial for establishing trust and hope as well as loosening the boundaries between patient and therapist, so a new intersubjective field can emerge, promoting empathy and understanding. Chapter 3, explicating the *resonant/relational imagination*, is closely related and explores the use of unconscious and nonverbal communication in the dyad, sometimes even eerily when the dyad is separated in time and space.

Chapters 4 and 5 take a more biological turn. Chapter 4 discusses the neuropsychological factors underlying "aha" moments. These moments can interrupt an enactment, helping the therapist and patient emerge from rigid self-states, allowing a meaningful reformulation of issues. The author's hope is that a neuropsychological understanding will help identify the imaginative skills needed to foster "aha" moments. Chapter 5 discusses *adaptive imagination*, the ability to solve problems and meet changing circumstances in a creative and flexible manner. Humans are biologically primed to be creative, even on a cellular level. Our body frequently responds to challenges spontaneously and effectively. Evolutionary processes are also considered and how they model an adaptive approach to problem-solving.

Embodied Imagination (EI), discussed in Chapter 6, is a specific technique of dreamwork in which the patient senses into dream images and embodies them. Expanding the imagination, this practice stimulates creativity and aids in problem-solving. It challenges the patient's habitual way of seeing the world and may facilitate the formation of new neural networks and new implicit memories. Using principles from chaos theory, EI builds a network of complex images and pushes this network to the edge of chaos so change can occur.

Trauma, discussed in Chapter 7, constricts the imagination and can damage any and all of these imaginative abilities. Meaning is transferred from the past to the present without transformation, creating rigid dysfunctional patterns and making it difficult to learn from experience. Creating artwork depicting trauma is discussed as an effective means of representing and resolving issues, as it provides an open space to work toward the transformation of disturbing traumatic memories. The struggle of the traumatized artist is also explored.

The *aesthetic imagination*, Chapter 8, continues to describe how various art forms – literature, theater, visual arts and architecture – can aid in healing. The artist brings his or her unconscious thoughts and feelings into the external world and in so doing transforms them (Bollas, 2011). As we experience a work of art, we participate in this transformation. The author's therapeutic experience in the Jewish Museum in Berlin outlines how experiencing a work of architecture can be healing.

Chapter 9, the final chapter, reviews the importance of surprise and containment, the need for the clinician and patient to find her voice, the value of the clinician listening to the hum in the ears[3] (her intuition), the inevitability of the patient himself deciding what he wants to be and the role of forgetting and remembering in trauma. The varieties of imagination are reprised.

Interestingly, as far back as the 12th century, Maimonides, Jewish philosopher, mystic and physician, emphasized the role of imagination in mental health and illness. For him, imagination can be positive and revelatory while other times, it can be misleading and create a disease of the soul, such as destructive behavior or mental disturbance. According to Maimonides, it is not ignorance but rather "disordered imagination" (Bakan et al., p. 50) that causes mental illness. Believing there should be physicians of the soul, Maimonides initiated a new approach to understand mental illness that ultimately influenced Sigmund Freud, who saw unconscious fantasies – the disordered imagination of Maimonides – as underlying neurosis (Bakan et al., 2009). In this sense, Maimonides' work can be viewed as the medieval precursor of psychotherapy and psychoanalysis.

Patients present with many varieties of trauma and disordered imagination. Examples range from the most extremely painful, such as victims of terror, to the more familiar: a relationship so "close" you cannot think your own thoughts or an authoritarian system of "rules" so suffocating you cannot dream. And let's not forget the everyday instance of the child who is so overscheduled he cannot even sense what he likes. While these situations differ in extremity, they have in common that the psyche is stifled and cannot perform what is a basic right: to dream and daydream and have the agency to execute and create what is uniquely one's own. Trauma can provoke affective numbing or overexcited hyperarousal, both of which limit freedom of expression. The traumatized individual may not have the emotional "space" to imagine.

Both Stephen Mitchell (1993) and Modell (1996) view psychopathology as a failure of the imagination, resulting in rigid self-states and the compulsive repetition of old patterns. To dissolve some of the rigidity, psychotherapists provide an atmosphere of listening that encourages the self to develop or be reclaimed. Dori Laub and Daniel Podell (1995) call this the restoration of the empathic other. Once the patient senses this, his imagination begins to be restored. Related, Phillip Bromberg (2013) writes that when the patient's capacity to transform fantasy into imagination increases, the imagined begins to feel possible. Agency is strengthened. Self-states can be negotiated smoothly, allowing the present and the future to be bridged.

In writing this book, I have used my intuition to anticipate the kinds of responses the reader may have – what reactions and questions she might pose in order to help expand her imagination. This expansion is necessary, not only to continuously improve the clinician's skill with patients but also to invent new ideas and symbols for the field, as symbols eventually get worn out and discarded (think penis envy, even the Oedipus myth and complex). Without the creation of new understandings, psychotherapy becomes tired and obsolete.

Viewing psychotherapy and imagination from many vantage points, each chapter of the book is meant to surprise the reader, to provide an enlivened space to provoke new thoughts and perspectives. The clinician may choose to give chapters to a patient for discussion and, hopefully, benefit. As a caveat, while I believe imagination and creativity can transform, I in no way diminish the challenge of change. This volume is meant to be an inspirational guide and companion in the very difficult, sometimes impossible, work of psychotherapy.

Imagination and creativity are frequently used nearly synonymously, exemplified by Winnicott (1985) and John Kaag (2008). On the other hand, a distinction can be made: imagination is the ability to think and feel flexibly and metaphorically so new connections can be made, while creativity is reserved for putting the imagination to use (Runco and Pina, 2013). From this perspective, imagination fuels creativity; however, in reality, one frequently blends with the other.

This volume explores how to live more "creatively" and also how to attempt creative work, such as writing an article for publication or using one's unconscious to comprehend a patient's struggle. This encompasses both types of creativity articulated by Mihaly Csikszentmihalyi (1996): (1) people who are personally creative, those who have a unique slant on life and find innovative solutions to problems and undertake creative activities but do not leave any actual creative work, as judged by the outside world. Everyday examples are a lawyer finding a solution to a thorny conflictual problem, a home chef preparing a really good meal or parents who meet the challenges of raising children in flexible and interesting ways and (2) people who are publicly creative who produce art that is objectively acclaimed by society, for example, Da Vinci, Michelangelo and Picasso. Arguably, the two categories overlap, as I view this second category more broadly than Csikszentmihalyi does. In terms of our field, this second category can include psychotherapists who publish, give presentations as well as do creative clinical work. Csikszentmihalyi stresses that to do creative work, one must have a domain, an area of expertise that one is mastering. All clinicians have that – the field of psychotherapy.

The use of discretion is important in creativity (Runco & Pina, 2013). For example, children need to learn when it is appropriate to be imaginative (that is, when to express themselves as individuals and when to conform and be conventional). This is consistent with research that indicates that an authoritative parenting style[4] is correlated with higher creativity in the child (Mehrinejad et al., 2015). Authoritative parenting is a flexible style characterized by warmth and moderate control. The reasons for the rules are frequently explained, such as how each person doing his chores helps the family function well as a unit. Recognizing the individuality of the child, the authoritative parent supports flexibility and change, therefore allowing variations to occur, but also provides structure and clear expectations (Baumrind, 1966, 1991). This approach facilitates the development of ego strength and self-discipline as well as independence of thought. These children learn to utilize imagination and are more likely to take it to a mature and practical level, the result being creative activity and accomplishment.

A *balance* of support and tension (family members are close but also separate) facilitates both positive mental health and high levels of development of creativity (Csikszentmihalyi et al., 1993). These families provide an environment for children that is both integrated (the family is supportive of one another) and differentiated (high expectations for children to develop their talents and strong encouragement of independent thought). This supports Diana Baumrind's classification of authoritative parenting as a positive style; authoritative parents do precisely what Csikszentmihalyi et al. stress: Children are integrated yet differentiated in these families.

Many patients have not yet learned this balance. They may overly conform and therefore have lost the sense of life's meaning or they are too idiosyncratic and unable to conform when it is in their best interest. Psychotherapy addresses this imbalance by providing an authoritative mix of independence and rules. The therapist encourages freedom of thought and expression yet still requires conforming to the rules of the frame, such as arriving on time, length of session and payment required.

The fourth goal is to experiment with interdisciplinary thinking to create a novel slant or innovative approach, including new ways to understand the basic questions psychotherapists face: how to help patients work through trauma, find hope and meaning, facilitate change of dysfunctional patterns, and foster adaptive problem-solving and emotional evolution. Creativity research has shown the value of the cross-fertilization of ideas across domains (Sill, 1996; Nissani, 1997; Ambrose, 2009; Jones, 2010). With this in mind, I explore and integrate ideas from many fields – biology and neuroscience, language and literature, architecture and design, biblical studies and mysticism.

The emphasis on interdisciplinary thinking is aimed at exploring metaphorical connections. Metaphor is evocative and creates a dynamic process in the reader. The poetic language of metaphor can awaken, stir and even alarm the imagination (Bollas, 1980, reviewing the work of Robert Rogers on metaphor). Understanding a process in another field may help activate fruitful, creative links with psychotherapy.

The imagination is based on metaphor. As Modell (2006, p. 27) writes, "Metaphor not only *transfers* meaning between different domains, but by means of novel recombinations, metaphors can *transform* meaning and generate new perceptions. Imagination could not exist without this recombinatory metaphoric process." The open and fluid use of metaphor is necessary for the free flow of the imagination. A well-known example is the chemist August Kekulé who discovered the closed carbon ring structure of organic compounds from a dream of twisting structures making snake-like motions. Suddenly one of the snake-like creatures seized its own tail, forming a ring, serving as a metaphor for the closed carbon ring. Kekulé awoke with a start and spent the rest of the night working out his hypothesis.

Interdisciplinary exploration is a form of cross-training for the brain. Viewing psychotherapy from many vantage points – spirituality, the arts and biology – increases flexibility of thought, provides new perspectives and suggests fresh approaches, all of which strengthen the imagination. The story of Adam and Eve typifies how interdisciplinary thinking can stimulate and arouse. According to Zornberg (1995), the story of Adam and Eve is a myth about desire, about wanting something that is absent. In the Midrashic literature[5] God desires something of human beings, simply that they should desire him. Desire also leads to consciousness and, eventually, maturity.

In the beginning, man is in a state of innocence and has no desire. Everything is perfect; to experience desire, something must be lacking. The serpent then seduces Eve to feel desire and eat fruit from the tree of knowledge. One interpretation is that God himself set the stage: by sending the snake and having Eve and Adam eat from the apple, then expelling them so they can move toward desire, experience and consciousness (Fromm, 1966; Aron, 2005). Desire enlivens consciousness and pushes one to strive and become more complete. Consciousness helps order and balance the experience of desire, so it does not overwhelm.

With patients, we recapitulate part of this story. We provide a kind of bliss in our close therapeutic relationship. (Is this our form of seduction?) We also usher in the exploration of incompleteness – what may be lacking – and the development of agency to fulfill desire. We see the value of the messy world as this creates desire, instead of the frequently fantasized world of perfection some patients crave, a world which will lack desire. The incompleteness that leads to desire is necessary for us to become more complete.

Finally, the fifth goal, this volume offers considerations about space for the reader to ponder: collapsed space with nowhere to think; transitional space where creativity and imagination reside; mystical space generating a restorative sense of oneness; actual physical space becoming potential, healing space; dramatic space, such as in therapeutic theater; and open, hopeful space in artwork addressing trauma (Laub and Podell, 1995).

Think of the space between reader and author, the therapist's sacred office space, quantum space (an object can be at two places at once!), infinite space; also, of course, foreclosed, narrow, barren, frenzied space – where many traumatized patients live.

I offer the reader space to reflect, to daydream, to remember; space to pursue goals, to make new connections; space to take risks and space to be wrong. Visiting these psychic and/or physical spaces helps both clinician and patient stretch and explore new ways of being in the world.

Notes

1 This is a time-limited eight-session therapy designed to work on a particular problem, according to the technique of Embodied Imagination (EI). It begins with an incubation (described in Chapter 6). This usually involves working a memory related to the problem as a dream, which then facilitates subsequent relevant dreams. These are worked according to the EI method.

2 This is a play on De Tocqueville's phrase: self-interest rightly understood, meaning that man serves himself by serving others or self-interest coincides with the

interest of the group (De Tocqueville, 1835/2004). With the real self, one's inside self can coincide, to a great extent, with one's outside self. Inner needs correspond to one's actions in the world.

3 The "hum in the ears" is a phrase Zornberg (1995, p. xix) uses to describe the beginning of a creative act with particular reference to Nadezhda Mandelstam's account of how her husband, renowned Russian poet Osip Mandelstam, would begin a new poem.

4 Authoritative parenting is to be distinguished from two other types of parenting, authoritarian and permissive (Baumrind, 1966, 1991). While authoritative parenting balances freedom and control, authoritarian parenting values obedience and expects orders to be obeyed without question. Authoritative parents tend to convince their children to follow family rules, while authoritarian parents regard their right to assert control as more important than their children's autonomy. On the other hand, permissive parents are lenient and tend to regard parental control as counterproductive to their children's development. They do not see themselves as responsible for shaping the child's ongoing or future behavior, while authoritative parents believe that it is important to guide their children and teach self-discipline and values. Succinctly, in authoritarian parenting, the power is vested in the parent, while in permissive parenting, the power is in the child. In authoritative parenting, there is a two-way balance; the parent is in charge but recognizes the individual interests of the child, encourages give and take and allows reasonable autonomy.

5 Midrashic literature refers to a type of Judaic biblical interpretation. It is a method that goes beyond the literal to establish the deeper meaning of the text, including using parable and allegory.

References

Ambrose, D. (2009). *Expanding visions of creative intelligence: An interdisciplinary exploration.* Cresskill, NJ: Hampton Press.

Aron, L. (2005). The tree of knowledge: Good and evil conflicting interpretations. *Psychoanalytic Dialogues*, 15:681–707.

Bakan, D., Merkur, D. & Weiss, D.S. (2009). *Maimonides' cure of souls: Medieval precursor of psychoanalysis.* Albany: State University of New York.

Baumrind, D. (1966). Effects of authoritative parental control on child behavior. *Child Development*, 37(4):887–907.

Baumrind, D. (1991). The influence of parenting style on adolescent competence and substance use. *Journal of Early Adolescence*, 11(1):56–95.

Bollas, C. (1980). Metaphor: A psychoanalytic view. *International Review of Psycho-Analysis*, 7:117–119.

Bollas, C. (Ed.) (2011). Creativity and psychoanalysis. In *The Christopher Bollas reader* (pp. 194–206). New York: Routledge.

Bosnak, R. (2018). *Inviting creative genius into your life.* Webinar, Jung Platform. February 1, 2018–June 28, 2018.

Bromberg, P.M. (2013). Hidden in plain sight: Thoughts on imagination and the lived unconscious. *Psychoanalytic Dialogues*, 23:1–14.

Carroll, L. (2015). *Alice's adventures in wonderland and through the looking glass.* New York: Barnes and Noble.

Csikszentmihalyi, M. (1996). *Creativity: Flow and the psychology of discovery and invention.* New York: Harper Collins.

Csikszentmihalyi, M., Rathunde, K. & Whalen, S. (1993). *Talented teenagers: The roots of success and failure.* Cambridge, UK: Cambridge University Press.
De Tocqueville, A. (1835/2004). *Democracy in America: The complete and unabridged volumes I and II.* New York: Random House.
Fromm, E. (1966). *You shall be as gods: A radical interpretation of the Old Testament and its tradition.* New York: Holt, Rinehart & Winston.
Jones, C. (2010). Interdisciplinary approach – Advantages, disadvantages, and the future benefits of interdisciplinary studies. *ESSAI (College of DuPage)*, 7(1):76–81.
Kaag, J. (2008). The neurological dynamics of the imagination. *Phenomenology and the Cognitive Sciences*, 8:183–204.
Kahr, B. (1996). *D. W. Winnicott: A biographical portrait.* Madison, CT: International Universities Press.
Kanter, J. (Ed.). (2004a). *Face to face with children: The life and work of Clare Winnicott.* London: Karnac.
Kanter, J. (2004b). "Let's never ask him what to do": Clare Britton's transformative impact on Donald Winnicott. *American Imago*, 61(4):457–481.
Laub, D. & Podell, D. (1995). Art and trauma. *International Journal of Psycho-Analysis*, 76:991–1005.
Mehrinejad, S.A., Rajabimoghadamb, S. & Tarsafic, M. (May 14–16, 2015). The relationship between parenting styles and creativity and the predictability of creativity by parenting styles. 6th World Conference on Psychology Counseling and Guidance, Antalya, Turkey.
Mitchell, S. (1993). *Hope and dread in psychoanalysis.* New York: Basic Books.
Modell, A. (1996). *Other times, other realities: Toward a theory of psychoanalytic treatment.* Cambridge, MA: Harvard University Press.
Modell, A. (2006). *Imagination and the meaningful brain.* Cambridge, MA: MIT Press.
Modell, A. (April 13, 2008). The unconscious as a knowledge processing center. 28th Annual Spring Meeting of the Division of Psychoanalysis (39) of the American Psychological Association, *Knowing, Not Knowing and Sort-of-Knowing: Psychoanalysis and the Experience of Uncertainty*, New York City, NY.
Nissani, M. (1997). Ten cheers for interdisciplinarity: The case for interdisciplinary knowledge and research. *The Social Science Journal*, 34(2):201–216.
Rodman, F.R. (2003). *Winnicott: Life and work.* New York: Da Capo Press.
Runco, M.A. & Pina, J. (2013). Imagination and personal creativity. In M. Taylor (Ed.), *The Oxford handbook of the development of the imagination* (pp. 379–386). New York: Oxford University Press.
Sill, D.J. (1996). Integrative thinking, synthesis, and creativity in interdisciplinary studies. *The Journal of General Education*, 45(2):129–151.
Winnicott, D.W. (Ed.) (1985). Communicating and not communicating leading to a study of certain opposites. In *The maturational process and the facilitating environment* (pp. 179–192). New York: International Universities Press.
Zelnick, L. (2014). Narrative surprise: Relational psychoanalytic process and biblical text. *DIVISION/Review*, 9:33–35.
Zornberg, A. (1995). *The beginnings of desire: Reflections on Genesis.* New York: Schocken Books.

Chapter 2

Spirituality and the imagination[1]

Psychotherapy is a sacred act, an I/Thou[2] experience conducted in sacred emotional and physical space. With respect and attentiveness, we listen to our patients in a special way, unconscious to unconscious, and cocreate a Third[3] space, in which old wounds can heal and new possibilities emerge. This listening requires us to use our deep imagination as we free-associate to our patient's communications and register our emotional and bodily responses. Our physical office is sacred as well, Jung's concept of temenos – an inviting presence, a secure containment, a home for the unconscious – where the work of psychotherapy can take place.[4]

Addressing the gradual lessening of boundaries in the therapeutic dyad, Bromberg (2013, p. 5) describes how patient and analyst grow more intersubjectively connected: "the miracle of right hemisphere 'creativity' slowly emerges within and between them – a shared process that makes each person feel 'larger' than before." This begins the entrance into transitional space, the land of imagination, originally described by Winnicott (1971), where we can dissolve internal rigidities and begin to connect with ourselves, with others and with the world. Containing an implicit spirituality, this is a feeling state located between external reality and inner psychic reality. By implicit spirituality I do not necessarily mean religious. In psychotherapy, implicit spirituality refers to the deep connection between patient and therapist that fosters our faith in the psychotherapeutic process. Entering this imaginal space helps the patient see beyond the literal, tolerate paradox and ambiguity and become more flexible and fluid. The imagination can transform, and this is deeply spiritual.

Considering spirituality and imagination synonymous, Jungian psychoanalyst and writer James Hillman (1992) views the spiritual world (soul/psyche) as a *perspective*; we use our imagination to view the world through a metaphorical lens. We see, as William Blake wrote, not just *with* the eyes (meaning literally) but also *through* the eyes (metaphorically). This includes dreams, images, fantasies and reflections. Hillman criticizes psychologies that are distant from the soul or psyche and therefore from the imagination.

Also linking imagination and spirituality, the poet W.H. Auden writes that the only concern of Primary imagination[5] is with sacred beings and events. We cannot anticipate these happenings; they must be encountered. And when they are, we are filled with awe. This reminds us of "moments of meeting" (Stern et al., 1998), unplanned moments in psychotherapy where there is an intense connection, beyond words, perhaps producing awe on both sides of the therapeutic dyad.

Throughout this volume, I will refer to bible stories, religious rituals and mystical beliefs not to endorse any particular religion or doctrine but for their poetry and metaphorical allusions to the psychotherapeutic process. Although I have favored stories from Judaism, as this is the tradition I know, I value and honor all traditions and welcome and enjoy commentary about their interpretations, customs and rituals, all of which can cast valuable light on the psychotherapeutic process (see especially, Hoffman, 2011).

But for now, come with me to the Museum for African Art in New York City to a stirring exhibit called "Facing the Mask." Let me introduce you to the world of masks and maskers. The maskers are fanciful presences that mediate between the secular and spiritual world and bring this knowledge to the people of the tribe. The word "mask" refers to a full-body costume that the person or "masker" assumes, usually very colorful, spectacular and otherworldly looking. One was a facemask buried in a haystack-shaped cloak of dried banana leaves, looking like a parade float. Ritual and ceremonial masks are an essential feature of the traditional culture of the peoples of a part of sub-Saharan Africa.

The masker must prepare himself for this sacred ritual. Before donning the mask, he undergoes a rite of passage for containing the soul of the dead, the ancestral spirit or force the mask represents. This involves an imaginative understanding of the religious and social functions of masking, an embodiment of the ancestral spirits and sometimes the use of substances aimed at inducing possession while still retaining some cognitive skills. (Sounds like a lot more fun than our psychoanalytic training institutes!) This is a performance-based art. The masker performs complicated movements and acrobatics – dancing, spinning, flying and dashing – as he or she creates the magic.

As spiritual leaders, the maskers help the members of the community enter transitional space to facilitate solving problems, settling disputes and moving from one developmental stage to another, from birth to death, and then even after. In the Dan peoples, near the Ivory Coast, the maskers are seen as supernatural beings who facilitate communication between people, including with their ancestors. To help with mourning, they drive the spirit of the deceased to the ancestral world so the living can return to life. As I viewed this exhibit, I realized how much therapists help patients transport themselves, whether from despair to hope, from stagnation to creativity, from reality to fantasy, or, as in the example above, vice versa.

Depending on the tribe, the maskers may have widely differing stylistic and conceptual approaches. However, just as in our field, there is also considerable overlap, as one tribe borrows a characteristic it likes from a neighboring tribe and incorporates it. Below you will see broad allusions to ongoing dialogues in psychotherapy. How inclusive can we be? How transparent are our methods? How much overlap between schools of thought?

In the Yoruba of Nigeria, one type of mask (*Engungun*) represents the recalling of ancestors from the dead to help with the sick and needy, resolve family disputes and facilitate the general well-being of the tribe. These ceremonies are shrouded in secrecy. The masks parade through the streets at night; the people have a curfew and must draw their shades so that the maskers can proceed in complete darkness. The night becomes a shroud for deepening the mysteries underlying the belief in reincarnation. The darkness shields the divine.

Another kind of mask (*Gelede*) is more open in its practices. Many times, it is literally transparent; the onlooker can see the person behind the mask. The goal of these ceremonies is to promote peace and harmony, and encourage all members of a community to interact with one another as children of the same mother. This ritual is open to women, whereas the previous one is not. In both ceremonies, the masker creates an atmosphere that allows the members of the tribe to feel intensely connected to facilitate healing.

The question of how and why the masks work remains a subject of scholarly debate. However, they are generally thought of as religious tools used as intermediaries between the world of the living and the supernatural universe. Masks summon spirits from the other world to perpetuate traditions or to introduce new religious, social or economic ideas (Herreman, 2002). From a psychotherapeutic perspective, the masker creates a play space through the use of imagery and fantasy to encourage the working through of issues and acceptance of new ideas. He or she is a guide in whom the community has deep faith; this helps the people lower their defenses, work through conflict and trauma and use their imagination to transform.

Maskers perform a public spiritual function but overlap with what I am viewing as our private, implicit spiritual function. Broadly speaking, one can think of the psychotherapist as the masker. When she assumes the "costume," she becomes a vessel, a mediator helping with communication with internalized objects (ancestors) from the past and the travel back and forth between conscious and unconscious processes. Just as the masker creates an atmosphere to foster the imaginative resources of the tribe, so too the therapist creates a sense of imaginative potential for the patient as she ushers him into transitional space, facilitating a feeling of trust and openness, operating in the zone where the strict boundaries of I/You dissolve. This is the area of faith (Eigen, 1981) where psychic healing takes place.

The Kabbalah and psychotherapy

In a seminal work, *Repair of the soul: Metaphors of transformation in mysticism and psychoanalysis*, Karen Starr (2008) explores Kabbalah to gain a deeper understanding of psychic change in psychoanalysis. The teachings of Kabbalah include a profound, mystical reshaping of the story of creation. It describes a partnership between God and humanity working together to create the world. God's motive for creating the world was a desire to be acknowledged, to be in relationship with human beings. In this process, not only are we transformed but we transform God – metaphorically echoing the relational dyad in psychotherapy in which patient and therapist deeply affect, at times transform, each other (Starr, 2008).

In Kabbalah, God represents deep structure while man represents surface (Arthur Green, 1999, as reported in Starr, 2008). In our terms, this suggests latent/manifest, implicit/explicit and unconscious/conscious. Just as patients work to find their true or authentic self, students of Kabbalah work to connect with this deeper structure by knowing themselves fully and authentically. This develops the divine spark or godliness within, which is at first hidden from consciousness. It is told that the 18th century Hasidic master Rabbi Zusya of Hanipol (Ukraine) declared before his death, "In the coming world, they will not ask me: 'Why were you not Moses?' They will ask me 'Why were you not Zusya?'" (Buber, 1991, p. 251, as quoted in Starr, 2008, p. 13). Similarly, we work in therapy to help the patient find his whole (holy) self.

Related, one of the great Jewish scholars of the 20th century, Rabbi Joseph Soloveitchik (1983) writes that it is man's sacred obligation to create, whether in repairing the flawed world or in actualizing his divine self. This viewing of creation and transformation as a religious act can serve as an analogy for understanding psychotherapy as a spiritual endeavor (Aron, 2005).

To help the patient find his authentic self, psychotherapy provides an immediate sense of union with another presence, allowing patient and therapist to operate, as mentioned above, in the area of faith, defined by Michael Eigen (1981, p. 413) as "a way of experiencing which is undertaken with one's whole being, all out, 'with all one's heart, with all one's soul, and with all one's might.'" It is to be fully immersed and alive.

The lessening of boundaries as the therapeutic dyad enters transitional space is related to the Kabbalistic description of the mystical, as follows. We are small circles within the large circle of God. At times the boundaries of our circle dissolve and then we have a mystical experience. At these moments, we are not *praying to* God; rather, we *participate with* God. We become at one with the divine. As part of this greater whole, we are released from the confines of ordinary reality and enter the space of potential transformation. Patient and therapist also become part of a greater whole, a cocreated Third. The dyad is safe to explore and imagine. With imagination we begin to create; in the Kabbalistic sense, this is an echo of God's creation of the world.

Reflecting on the power of deep emotional connection, Martin Buber, a philosopher, theologian and Hassidic scholar, defines two types of relations: I/Thou and I/It (Buber, 1970). The I/Thou is a spiritual, living relationship where both members are subjects and share a unity of being. Each person is able to imaginatively sense into the psyche of the other, becoming so closely connected that there are no discrete boundaries. This is not limited to people; it can be a relationship with a tree, a field of flowers, the sky or even a hammock in the backyard. The essence is that the distance between the other melts away, and the only important thing is the living, dialogic relationship – what we strive for in psychotherapy. The I/It relationship, on the other hand, is detached. Each member is discrete and separate; each is an object to the other.

There is an apocryphal story that one day when Buber was busy at his desk arranging papers for an upcoming lecture, a young rabbinical student came in and clumsily told him about his concerns. Buber answered perfunctorily, not really listening. As soon as the student left, Buber went back to his work. Tragically, the student committed suicide shortly afterward. Realizing he and the student had been in an I/It relationship, very separate from each other, Buber vowed at that moment to listen intently and deeply in the future. He would create what he termed an I/Thou relationship with others, an echo of man's relationship with God.

A colleague reminded me of the value of deep connection as he described the strong solidarity among the men he consults with in a firehouse since 9/11. This is larger than any one man and intensely felt by all – many of the men report religious experiences, even visions. These men participate in the intermediate realm of intense connectedness, and this may give them the fortitude to face the unpredictable, frightening nature of their world as well as provide a deep sense of belonging and meaning.

In a similar vein, Janet Sayers (2002), in an article about the psychoanalyst Marion Milner, refers to the mystical elements of working in the area of faith when one experiences the immediate sense of union with another presence. Milner emphasizes the potential for health and creativity in overcoming resistance to the mystical experiences of oneness, which she sometimes calls the unconscious or the id or God. I would reword this as an experience of coming close to the deepest parts of oneself and/or connecting deeply to something outside the self, whether it be a fully immersed relationship with another person, one's work, nature or simply a sense of the underlying harmony of the universe. Aspects of these issues pervade psychotherapeutic work through the reciprocally deep, implicitly spiritual connections present in the therapeutic dyad.

The Kabbalist myth of creation

Based on the teachings of Isaac Luria (1534–1572), the Lurianic Kabbala provides a creation myth with which to imagine psychotherapy, a myth with a relational perspective. In this vein, Kerry Gordon (2004) views aspects of relational psychoanalysis as a modern creation myth, "intended in part to foster psycho-spiritual regeneration through the repair of our broken capacity for sacred experience" (Gordon, 2004, p. 12).

The Kabbalist creation myth embraces dialectics: *alienation/construction, deconstruction/restoration and exile/redemption*. When God created the world, he stepped back or contracted, creating a void to make space for the world (alienation). When He proclaimed, "Let there be light" (Gen. 1:3), primordial light filled the darkness. This light, His divine attributes or sefirot,[6] shone forth and came down in vessels (construction). These became the potential attributes of man: will/desire, wisdom, understanding, kindness, judgment, beauty, endurance, splendor, foundation and kingship (Drob, 2000; Starr, 2008).

However, the vessels were not able to contain the divine light and shattered into shards (deconstruction). While some light returned to its divine source to begin a process of repair, some fell below into the empty space and attached itself to the broken shards. This formed husks, lifeless shells but with a divine inner core of light, giving energy to the shells. From this power, the husks create the lower worlds, including the world of evil. All mankind is now thrust into exile. These lower worlds are filled with moral, spiritual and psychological contradictions but also are the source of ultimate redemption. Our charge is to continue the repair of the world by gathering up all the divine light and all the souls imprisoned as a result of the trapped light (restoration). The vessels will then be repaired, the light returned to its Divine source and the world redeemed (Drob, 2000; Schwartz, 2007; Starr, 2008).

These themes are present in psychotherapeutic work. The patient frequently comes to us feeling alienated and anxious, shattered and in a state of exile. His desires may be repressed or his self-states dissociated. He may feel imprisoned by a false self. If the therapeutic process goes well, the patient's dissociation or repression lessens. He becomes more whole, and his divine inner core (true self) begins to flourish. This is psychological redemption (Drob, 2000). As we help the patient leave the imprisonment of dysfunctional patterns, we are performing a sacred mission. We are repairing the world.

Free will and the void

The Kabbalistic creation myth offers hope. God contracts to make room for the world and honor our separate reality. Therefore, we have free will and the capacity to repair the world and even transform God. But how does this happen?

The interesting metaphor of God as "author" of the Bible is considered in an interview of Avivah Zornberg by Krista Tippet (October 6, 2011). Just as an author loses control of his characters (the characters come to have lives of their own), so too God loses control of us. Zornberg clarifies that it:

> ... is not exactly losing control. It's actually discovering forces that were not explicit before ... and suddenly ... these forces and these ways of creating things suddenly become real. So in that sense, it's losing control in terms of a neat, unmessy package.

In this metaphor, God acts as a good psychotherapist. He or She tolerates the messiness of allowing these implicit forces to emerge to bring about creation and change. He or She learns in the process and teaches us how to learn.

Turning to the traditional biblical story of creation, Adam and Eve were punished, banished for eating from the Tree of Knowledge and thrown into the unknown. Yet without this knowledge, how could they ever have free will? How could they ever "know" God and transform Him in the process of repair? Before they ate the apple, Adam and Eve were in complete bliss, almost robotlike, without desire or agency. Only after they leave Eden and gain consciousness can they begin the long process of repair and possibly begin to comprehend God as well. As detailed by Lewis Aron (2005), Eric Fromm even raised the possibility that God arranged for the serpent to seduce Eve so the first couple would leave the bliss of Eden and gain maturity and consciousness.

This seeming contradiction of void as emptiness and void as potential is well known to students of Kabbalah. A void is necessary for creation – both for God to create the world and for Adam and Eve to develop desire, agency and free will. In psychotherapy, the therapist also needs to step back (contract) to make room for the patient and his or her desire. The patient might have to endure emptiness and messiness to imagine and create new possibilities. And both patient and therapist need to be in a continuous process of uncertainty (another type of void) as they learn how to learn.

In fact, one interpretation is that the Kabbalists view the void or darkness (*ayin*) as closer to the divine than the light, as before creation there was only the Divine *Ayin*, closer in meaning to divine potential. In Hebrew, *ayin*, void or darkness, is usually contrasted with *yesh*, meaning something or being. In the beginning, God contracts to create a void so His light can form the world. It is out of this void that "something" is created. However, for some Kabbalists, creation is *not* something arising out of nothing but rather the emergence of all existence from the supreme hidden source of existence, the divine *Ayin*.

Psychotherapy, the process of creating from *ayin*, recognizes this divine potential in the patient. Out of the darkness of not-knowing comes knowing.

Out of formlessness comes form. Out of chaos comes order. As the dyad surrenders to the unknown, *Ayin* is reframed as pure potential; from this comes emotional understanding and action for change. This is the Kabbalistic paradox: out of nothing (in the most profound sense of pure potential) comes being.[7]

Bion and Kabbalah

In my view, a poet foremost and psychoanalyst second, Bion's writings are particularly compatible with Kabbalistic thought (Bion, 1962, 1967, 1977, 1988). He viewed psychoanalysis, as well as mysticism and science, as a search for being at one with ultimate reality, as a search for O. Regarding psychotherapy or psychoanalysis, this is the meaning or emotional "truth" of the session. While this truth can never be fully known, with faith and intuition, the good therapist senses its presence. O, what some call the Godhead, is similar in meaning to the Kabbalists' word for God: *Ein-soph* (infinite or boundless) or *Ayin* (no-thing) and All (Starr, 2008).

In Bion's mystical exhortation to enter each psychoanalytic session without memory or desire (Bion, 1988), that is, to enter the void, he is facilitating the analyst's entrance into O, from which the analyst makes his interpretations. Predicated on an act of faith, transformation is facilitated when the patient enters O and has made the transition from "knowing" (intellectual understanding) to "being" (a new emotional understanding). Bion (1977) analogized his revolutionary work to the impact the Kabbalist Luria had on the traditional rabbinate, which was seen by the Kabbalists as overly intellectual and rule bound (Starr, 2008).

To bring the psychotherapeutic data to consciousness, the therapist uses his (spiritual) imagination to "dream" the session so that the patient's fragmented thoughts (beta elements) can be re-presented (alpha elements) in a usable form.[8] To accomplish this, the therapist empties himself, much like the mystic. The therapist must accept this void, the formlessness of the beginning of the session, and not formulate prematurely. Then something will come out of "nothing." This is what it means to be in the present moment, as memory is the past and desire is the future. The therapist must pay the kind of wide attention that is like religious contemplation, what Bion terms a state of reverie.

Reverie is a concentrated form of the free-floating attention advocated by Freud. For Bion, the analyst's reverie, a state of extreme receptivity, is modeled on the original mother (caretaker)/infant relationship. The attuned mother processes the infant's unmetabolized mental states and bodily sensations. Through her words and actions, the mother calms the child and communicates her understanding. When this is successful, the child's overwhelmed states become manageable, and ultimately, he is able to self-regulate.

A similar process occurs with the psychotherapist. In her reverie which facilitates access to unconscious communication, the therapist helps the patient translate inchoate thoughts into states of emotional understanding. In this state of reverie, the therapist may feel lost at times, and that is the correct feeling. As Bion's daughter, Parthenope Bion Talamo wrote, for Bion, analysis is the search for the truth, and truth is not an absolute but in a continuous process of becoming. This search is an ongoing journey: "... if you anchor yourself, you stop travelling" (Talamo, 2018, p. 4).

According to Bion, to be truly open to the sparks of truth, the analyst cannot control the emotional reality of a session, including the wish to "help" the patient. For Bion, the analyst's basic working orientation is the importance of perception and attention over memory and knowledge. The analyst's observations do not have to do with the past (memory) nor the future (desire) but with the immediacy of the moment. If the analyst is able to sustain faith in O and tolerate the development of formulations that reflect O, he may legitimately hope for a therapeutic outcome in which the patient becomes more at one with himself (Eigen, 1981).

Bion's work is inspirational and aspects of a psychoanalytic ideal. However, practically, his observations apply at certain times in the treatment while memory and desire have their place at others. Also, although Bion's is a two-person psychology, that is, what happens in the session is in the link between the analyst and patient and each influences the other, current thinking is focused less on the analyst/therapist formulating the emotional truth of the session, as Bion suggests, but rather in cocreating it with the patient. Finally, words like absolute truth and ultimate reality, in my understanding, also represent an ideal. As mentioned above, for Bion, the "truth" is always in a state of becoming. It is never absolute or immutable (Talamo, 2018).

Flow

The feeling of implicit spirituality in transitional experiencing is related to flow (Csikszentmihalyi, 1990, 1996), defined as complete absorption and energized focus, a feeling of timelessness, a sense of being outside everyday reality. We are part of a greater whole, larger than ourselves, which can catapult us into the sacred. This is similar to the area of faith described by Eigen (1981) and entrance into O by patient and analyst, as described by Bion.

Flow is a crucial and insufficiently appreciated characteristic of the creative process. When in this state and also involved in an area of high expertise, we are likely to be open and experimental and experience "aha" insights that can lead to innovation (Csikszentmihalyi, 1996), presuming that we follow up the insights with the very hard work needed to bring a particular project or activity to fruition.

In the "zone" of flow, we are able to function so well because we are totally focused, without the anxiety of being over– or understimulated. The artist Rachel Shapiro (Domash and Shapiro, 2012) describes her experience of flow as follows:

> Flow is a semi-trance like state where I enter a creative bubble and am able to truly release. In this space I achieve great focus and have fine attention to detail … I also let go of judgment of my work. The artwork happens, takes on a life of its own and begins to evolve. I facilitate its coming into being, its eruption, its various births and deaths. … There is extreme focus and solitude in my actions and paradoxically, although the world seems to fall away, there is also a strong sense that every brushstroke is interconnected in a beautiful and intricate fabric that makes up the universe. I experience the state of flow as a portal, a gateway, an opening. These entrances are invitations to go deeper and to peel back one more layer. This is a state to which I always want to return, sometimes feeling lost on an ever-changing path. How to return is a question I am constantly asking myself.

Shapiro's experience of flow allows her to be in the moment and also to move beyond, toward interconnectedness and potential transformation. She also manifests the anxiety of creation. Can and how do we return to this state?

In psychotherapy, as in artistic work, the sense of flow facilitates freedom from self-judgment, allowing for novel associations and expansion of the imagination. This can be corroborated neuropsychologically. Charles Limb and Allen Braun (2008) studied improvisation in relation to jazz musicians and found that the dorsolateral prefrontal cortex (DLPFC), responsible for monitoring one's performance, including self-censoring and inhibition, shuts down completely during improvisation while the medial prefrontal cortex (MPFC) increases in activity, an area that manages functions of attuned communication, empathy and intuition as well as activities that convey individuality.

Deactivation of the DLPRC may be associated with the kind of free-floating attention that permits spontaneous unplanned associations and sudden insights or realizations (Limb & Braun, 2008), that is, creative intuition may operate when an attenuated DLPRC no longer regulates the contents of consciousness, allowing unfiltered, unconscious or random thoughts and sensations to emerge. In this state there is a relative absence of anxiety. The authors explain that just as over-thinking a jump shot, that is, introducing self-monitoring brain mechanisms, can cause a basketball player to fall out of the zone and perform poorly, the opposite is also true. The dampening of self-monitoring brain mechanisms helps promote the free flow of novel ideas and impulses.

This may be the neural equivalent of how patient and therapist feel as a result of the positive therapeutic alliance; there is a sense of deep trust in the process, and affect is well regulated. This allows for a relaxation of judgment and criticality and an opportunity to experience new ways of being the world. There is a potential paradox here more fully explored in Chapter 4. At times, insight can also emerge from moments of high anxiety, such as during enactments when the dyad begins to feel a sense of pressure and urgency. It may be that under certain circumstances, anxiety, if not too overwhelming, can also help with intense focus (Lehrer, 2008) and can facilitate insights bursting through to consciousness.

Struggling with faith

When we fall out of flow, we fall "out of faith" – and faith is an important element of healing. In part, psychotherapists are relying on the placebo effect, a very real healing action that unfortunately has the negative connotation of being insignificant or confounding in research studies. However, a placebo can have powerful healing effects, as elaborated in Chapter 5. If one has faith in a treatment, it will frequently work (even when there is no treatment at all but the patient thinks there is). That is the power of faith.

In psychotherapy, patient and therapist dive deeply and hopefully into the process while containing and exploring doubts. Similarly, in the creative process, we must sustain faith in our project, while at the same time accepting doubt, even despair, along the way. This is the light mingled with darkness. Remember, the darkness may be simply shielding the light, as in Psalms 189:12, "The Divine Presence makes darkness its hiding place." Eventually, the light shines through.

Of course, sometimes patient and/or therapist struggle with a falling "out of faith." In a previous communication (Domash, 2009), I discussed the ordinary example of a new patient who expressed his lack of faith in psychotherapy – his skepticism, his feeling it is self-indulgent. He even retorts, "Why couldn't I just become a monk instead!" (He is possibly alluding to his spiritual needs.) Despite the patient's protests, I did see him actually begin to use the sessions to start to face his current crises (alcohol use, unemployment, marital problems). He would address these issues and then periodically return to his skepticism. While his cynicism is a form of resistance, he is also discussing the issue of faith: what to believe in, whom to trust and whether he can allow himself to hope.

Discussing the Exodus from Egypt, Zornberg (2015) describes the Jewish people's loss of faith as they wander through the desert trying to reach the Promised Land. At the demand of his doubtful people, Moses sends 12 spies to check out the Land to see if God has been truthful in his promise. God is not pleased that Moses accedes to these demands, although leaves the decision up to Moses. Riddled with insecurities, the spies return and give mixed messages. While acknowledging the Promised Land is very fertile, indeed, a land of "milk and honey," they report the inhabitants are very powerful with heavily fortified cities. Many are even giants – an idea that gets greatly exaggerated as they retell the story. In comparison, the spies themselves felt tiny and small, like "grasshoppers" (Num. 13:33) *and the inhabitants saw them as such.*

This only intensifies the Israelites' loss of faith and creates mass panic. Zornberg (2015) writes that the Israelites' intense anxieties cannot be fully accounted for by possible defeat in war. Rather, at their core, the Israelites are terrorized by the anticipation of seismic change, of being reborn as free men. This is analogous to so many of our patients who are frightened to leave old destructive patterns and create a new life.

Shocked and astonished by the Israelites' fears, Moses does nothing to calm the situation. In our terms, this is an enactment. The Israelites' panic triggers a loss of faith in Moses, and he becomes temporarily useless. Only Joshua and Caleb, the two spies who were optimistic, attempt to give the people hope.

God is very angry on several accounts. He allows the spies to have their fears, but when they begin to project these fears onto the inhabitants of the new Land, they go too far. The spies cannot presume to know what the inhabitants think. They cannot limit the imagination of the Other. God questions the projections of the spies: "Who told you that you didn't look like angels in their eyes?" (quoted from the Midrash Tanchuma[9] by Zornberg, 2015, p. 102). Zornberg (2015, p. 103) writes, "God is angered at their fatal constriction of imaginative possibility." This is a powerful example of how projection can limit possibilities. We are reminded how patients frequently seek confirmation of their fears, as the Israelites did.

Second, Moses now has a rebellion on his hands. The people are very frightened and cry out to choose a new leader to return to Egypt – attempting to reverse God's plan. Metaphorically, here we see the return of the repetition compulsion – in this case, enslavement to Pharaoh. As Zornberg (2015, p. 103) writes, "The wish to return to Egypt is the wish to be in the death place, at the end of imagination." It is more comfortable to go back into certain slavery, perhaps death, than face the danger of possible war and, more importantly, the fear of change and freedom.

God punishes this lapse of faith and loss of imagination. For the 40 days the spies journeyed to the Promised Land, the people spend 40 years wandering in the desert until the adult population dies out with the exception of the two men who had faith: Joshua and Caleb. No one who questioned God reaches the Promised Land. Led by Joshua, only their descendants can enter.

While this seems irrationally harsh, I take God's anger and subsequent punishment as a metaphor for the possible grave consequences when faith and imagination are lost. I have been repeatedly convinced that the ability to do good psychotherapeutic work or to create a work of art is, in part, a consequence of faith – even when we feel we are wandering in the wilderness. For example, if we start to lose faith in our work with a patient, we need to reflect and break through whatever paralysis is occurring. Hopefully then, the developing enactment will cease and our effective interaction with the patient restored. The same applies to writing this book. I must persevere with intention, even if I have no ideas that day or feel I am not writing well. I must have faith and imagine that if I continue working, I will reach my goal, my Promised Land.

I'd like to give you an account of my own loss of confidence, faith and hope in the aftermath of the terror of 9/11. Discouraged and frightened, I began to experience an inner emptiness. In my sense of loss, I did not realize a vastness was being created in me that I could fill. This is emptiness in a positive sense, emptiness as potential space – a fertile void, an *Ayin*, from which something new can emerge. Or as psychoanalyst James Ogilvie (2002, p. 2) challenges, "Can we in Wittgenstein's words 'let ourselves be struck?'"

My New York City office is close to Ground Zero. September 11 was my first day back after a long vacation of six weeks. A patient told me at 10 AM what was happening, as best he could tell. This began several days of terror and numbness. My husband had been standing in front of the Towers when the first one fell and literally ran ahead of the plume of smoke. If necessary, he was fully prepared to jump into the East River and swim to avoid what he thought was an enveloping explosion. Later that day, we began to realize that most phones were not working. People were afraid to use public transportation. Some subway lines were out. Others would go unpredictable routes. Bomb scares were rampant. I didn't know who was coming to sessions and who wasn't. Some patients did come, especially those who lived nearby. A police barricade was put up, not letting anyone south of 14th Street enter who was not a resident. (My office is on 12th Street.) I had to explain to police officers why they should let my patients go through the barricade.

Of course, in subsequent weeks and months, many patients were terrified and despairing. Particularly poignant were a number of patients who had struggled to immigrate from countries with political oppression and persecution, only now to feel persecuted here. Then patients started to lose jobs and medical insurance and slowly exited my practice. I tried to informally stay in touch with these people. Some would call from time to time; others would keep me informed by notes. When it helped, I reduced fees and frequency of sessions. No new referrals came in at all.

I began to feel anxious, irrelevant. Adding to this mix of gloom and despair were the ongoing terror warnings, their unpredictability. Then eight or nine months later, the stock market decline frightened people further. On a purely personal level, the second of my two children had recently gone off to college, and I was struggling with a very real void in the home.

I was beginning to lose my imagination.

I felt a shattering in the outside world and, to some extent, inside me. This makes it hard to have the inner strength and access to the unconscious needed to do really good psychodynamic psychotherapy. I felt I was losing my field of study and my practice. One thing that did help was to realize that my patients and I had been through the same trauma, the first time that had ever happened. I was able to join them and acknowledge their fears, perhaps in a way as never before.

I began to understand that it was not so much my field I was losing, as my own sense of productivity, creativity and imagination. I felt without vitality and ideas. I had no strong sense of a future. This is emptiness in our usual negative sense. Before I "knew." Now I knew nothing.

To stimulate my imagination, I began to read psychoanalytic and psychotherapy journals again. Prior to this, as I helped my two children prepare for and attend college, there had been little free time for reflection and reading. Now that my children had left, I could turn to a more thoughtful consideration of the field. As I read, I felt nourished by joining the thinking of colleagues. I began to feel connected and free to pursue many avenues of interest. I was reconnecting to an underlying sense of wholeness.

I had for a long time been interested in pursuing a new venture, apart from psychotherapy, that would allow me to chronicle personal philosophy in the form of helping people write "ethical wills." This had been an idea with no actualization. Shortly after 9/11, my husband heard a short piece on National Public Radio about a project like this. He excitedly told me about it, knowing this is what I wanted to do. I began imagining ways to actualize my ideas. I then became active in developing a program and setting up the infrastructure to do this. The vastness within me opened to this stroke of luck – the NPR program – and the idea took hold.

I see this as a fortuitous blend of imagination (or unconscious freedom) and luck. For the therapist or patient, unconscious freedom is the ability to work in the implicit or unconscious realm with empathy and creativity while being relatively free of anxiety. This kind of freedom can help one recognize an opportunity that can create change.

As I slowly began to find my vitality, I came across the work of an artist who uses leaves and flowers to make delicate yet forceful impressions with paint. She used the first new growths from Ground Zero and imaginatively made these into works of art. One of her prints is hanging in my home. Her work symbolizes revitalization and renewal.

How to enter transitional space with patients

How do we enter this flow state with patients? What kind of "dance" do we do?

Although we certainly are not always successful, we frequently are able to perform our psychotherapeutic ritual by attentive listening, by an unobtrusive stance (Grossmark, 2012), by nonverbal messages of acceptance, by our surrender to the process (Ghent, 1990), by imagining ourselves in the other (Sayers, 2002) and by "digesting" the patient's problems and returning poetic (when at our best) understanding (Bion, 1962). These methods foster trust and openness, allowing the damaged parts of the self to emerge and be repaired.

The unobtrusive analyst

In sensitive detail, Robert Grossmark (2012) describes how by offering the patient unobtrusive but companioning engagement, the analyst is not abstinent but deeply involved without being overwhelming. This is to be distinguished from aspects of the current relational approach that asks the patient to reflect on the intersubjective relationship and how the therapeutic experience is mutually constructed. For patients who may experience deadness and an inability to see the other as a separate person or who may not be able to reflect all, this approach can be shameful and retraumatizing. The "good-enough" analyst adjusts his technique accordingly and, in such a case, works slowly and carefully.

This is in the tradition of Michael Balint (1968) and Winnicott (1965). Balint describes patients who cannot use standard analytic technique and instead need a more primitive type of analytic relationship, a benign regression, which allows the most damaged aspects of the patient's self to emerge. This approach encourages thoughts and feelings, barely sensed, to take form (Winnicott, 1965). The patient is able to inscribe the analysis with his own individual stamp.

Grossmark describes how an unobtrusive approach is facilitated by quietness and patience. This is not the type of silence associated with the old concept of neutrality, now seen as "cold." Although remaining in the background, the unobtrusive analyst is still very much with the patient. Analogously, Thomas Ogden (2004, p. 95) writes how the mother's "unobtrusive presence provides a setting for the infant's constitution to begin to make itself evident, for development to unfold, for the infant to experience spontaneous movement and become the owner of his own sensations." The same holds true for the unobtrusive analyst and his patient.

This unobtrusive approach has value even with less traumatized patients, as it gives the patient needed space to develop. The gains from therapy are then more likely to be the patient's own rather than profundity offered by an "omniscient" analyst. As Grossmark reminds us, the analyst has to remember not to commit an unintentional "act of theft" (Ogden, 1989, p. 176) by wanting to connect so much with a patient that she unwittingly takes away the patient's ability to make a mark on his own therapy. Most psychotherapy would benefit from a mixture of a more active relational approach and a stepping back to a more unobtrusive but companionable stance.

This is reminiscent of the stepping back of God in the Kabbalistic myth of creation. He contracts (steps back) so the light can come in and create the world. Also, by giving up His omnipotent, all-embracing presence, His "*every-whereness*," He leaves space for the Other who has a separate reality and the possibility of free will (Winkler & Elior, 1994). The clinician, too, must know when to step back. Just as in the Kabbalistic creation myth, God honors us in our separate reality, so too the clinician must honor the patient in his.

The importance of surrender

Surrender has negative connotations in the West, usually indicating a display of weakness. But the meaning intended here is spiritual surrender, a "giving to" rather than a "giving up," a yielding rather than a submission. Facilitating an expansion of the self, this surrender involves a willingness to let down defensive barriers and, if necessary, a giving up of the false self (Ghent, 1990). This may necessitate a profound therapeutic regression. Winnicott (1975) describes such a case in which the patient surrendered her false caretaker self to him, her analyst, so she could access her true self and feel more free.

Surrender and regression are close, and reminiscent of Milner's emphasis on the healing power of regression and the importance for some patients to break down false inner organizations, which do not really belong to them. With the patient's surrender, we can more easily "find" him or her, as working with this type of patient can seem like a game of hide-and-seek. It's easier to play this game if there is some ability in both patient and therapist to experience a form of egoless surrender.

We surrender to become more whole and more known. Emmanuel Ghent (1990) points out that the words *healing, making whole* and *holy* all have the same linguistic derivation, again a linking of healing and spirituality. Quoting Erich Fromm, Ghent writes that the word "sin" in the Old Testament literally means "missing an opportunity to be present, alive" (Fromm, 1966, p. 132). The remedy is to surrender and access the true self in order to become fully present and whole (holy). Ghent (1990, p. 109) writes, "Faith, surrender, the beginnings of creativity and symbol formation all intersect in the world of transitional experiencing …."

The issue of surrender and healing is also addressed by Bromberg (2013). When the treatment is going well, patient and analyst surrender to the therapeutic process in several ways. First, they relax their grip on the self-states that previously defined the "truth" about each other. At the same time, they allow their own self-states to be less rigidly defended, as there is less need to defend against otherness. Both of these processes allow previously incompatible truths about the other to now coexist. This surrender creates a unity of being, which is healing. As such, this process can undo a creative block, which may be thought of as dissociated states that cannot be integrated into consciousness.

Potential physical space

While we have been focusing on emotional attunement, physical space can also encourage the development of potential space. As part of an ongoing project of photographing psychoanalysts in their offices, Mark Gerald (2011) writes about how we aim to secure a continuous containment for our patients and create a sacred physical space where we belong. Our offices become the holding environment for our work, a "house for the unconscious world" (Gerald, 2011, p. 436), a space where the darkest fears can be explored. Marion Woodman (2011), a Jungian analyst, also writes that the office should be cherishing and calm, a place away from the stresses of the workaday world – for example, quiet, peaceful and colorful images can be picked up by the patient from art in the room. For Woodman, the image is the connector between psyche and soma. The entire atmosphere of the office contributes to the ability of the dyad to be present in the moment and engage in authentic and meaningful connection.

Moving away from the privacy of the psychotherapist's office to the public world of architecture and design, I was very moved by my experience in The Jewish Museum of Berlin (Domash, 2014a,b), discussed more fully in Chapter 8. Long haunted by the Holocaust and stories of family members lost, I needed to travel to Berlin to experience this Museum. In Kabbalistic terms, during my visit, the boundaries between the physical museum and the edges of myself blurred. I felt an intense emotional connection to the surround and, by extension, to the architect Daniel Libeskind. This experience connected me to my mother and grandmother, both long passed away. They lived in America during the War but desperately feared for many of their relatives still living in Europe. Their relatives were all incarcerated and, in many cases, killed. Libeskind's brilliantly artful and thoughtful design was able to both contain and reveal this horror and transport me to transitional space so I could process it.

Therapeutic use of hallucinogenics to achieve a mystical state

The value of experiencing mystical/spiritual feelings in psychotherapy is starkly demonstrated by the recent, renewed clinical interest and research in the hallucinogenic psilocybin, the active ingredient in magic mushrooms. Several studies (Griffiths et al., 2008, 2011, 2016; Ross et al., 2016) have demonstrated that a single psychedelic experience, in conjunction with follow-up psychotherapy, can have profound, long-lasting mental health benefits. The 2016 studies referenced are the most rigorously controlled to date.

The subjects of the research are patients who had been experiencing intense anxiety subsequent to a cancer diagnosis. As a result of taking psilocybin, they had a psychedelic experience that stimulated mystical/spiritual feelings. The patients' symptoms were greatly reduced, including decreases in cancer-related demoralization and hopelessness, improved spiritual well-being and increased quality of life. The researchers concluded that the psilocybin-induced mystical experience brought about the therapeutic effect, and that the effect may last for as long as eight months postdosing. Further, they indicated a single dose leading to both immediate and long-lasting antidepressant and antianxiety effects is novel in psychiatry. Just how the therapeutic effect is achieved is the subject of future research (Ross et al., 2016).

While psilocybin can create feelings of relaxation and mystical, spiritual experiences, it can also create nervousness, paranoia and panic. However, the researchers did not report any negative effects with the use, possibly because of the supportive therapeutic atmosphere. The subjects took their small dose in a calm, peaceful room where they also had their therapy sessions. The therapist was present; there was music playing.

While the researchers in the above studies do not speculate on the biological mechanisms underlying mystical experiences, researchers at the Imperial College in London (Tagliazucchi et al., 2014) have undertaken studies that suggest that psilocybin synchronizes brain activity in areas related to emotion and memory, resembling a wakeful state of dreaming. According to the researchers, this may help explain the psychedelic effects of psilocybin which include unconstrained cognition, hyperassociation, and changes in the subjects' perception of time, space and selfhood. In my view, it is reasonable that these characteristics facilitate an expansion of consciousness and mystical experiencing.

Further, these studies illuminate the interpenetration of imagination and spirituality. Katherine MacLean et al. (2011) studied the effects of psilocybin on personality of the patients who experienced mystical experiences. They found that these subjects had significantly more openness for up to one year after the single administered dose. Openness is a personality trait that includes aesthetic appreciation and sensitivity, imagination and fantasy, and tolerance for differing viewpoints and values. This may suggest related pathways for both mystical experiences and imagination.

End thoughts

Whether as metaphorical masker or Kabbalistic guide, the therapist facilitates the patient's entrance into transitional space, a sacred spiritual space where transformation is possible. This is foundational in helping the dyad reach deep levels of unconscious communication, a process which can create change. As the boundaries between patient and therapist become more semipermeable, each may begin to know the other better than the other knows him or herself. This sensing into the other's psyche can reach an uncanny level at times – the subject of our next chapter. Some explanations follow ....

Notes

1 Parts of this chapter appeared in an earlier version in Domash (2009) and are gratefully reprinted with permission from Guilford Press.
2 Articulated by theologian Martin Buber (1970), the concept of I/Thou describes the essence of a sacred living relationship. The boundaries between self and other fall away and the only thing important is the relationship with the other. This ultimately brings one closer to God or the Eternal Thou and the meaning of life. God is the ultimate Thou for Buber.
3 Ogden (1994) discusses the analytic third as the jointly created unconscious life of the analytic pair, which gives space for freedom of expression and imaginative development. In his view, an essential aspect of analysis involves the analyst tracking the movement back and forth between the individual subjectivity of the patient and analyst and their joint intersubjectivity. These exist in tension with each other just as the mother and infant are both joined and separate, as they "create, negate and preserve the other" (Ogden, 1994, p. 4).
4 See Gerald (2011, p. 245) for an extensive discussion of the meaning of our work space and the importance of "finding a space where we can belong, with our belongings, …"
5 Primary imagination, a term used by the romantic poets, is defined by Samuel Coleridge as the power of perception. Operating at an unconscious level, primary imagination makes it possible to form images and know things. Coleridge viewed the primary imagination of humans as an echo of God's acts of creation. Secondary imagination differs in degree but not in kind from primary imagination. Coming from both the conscious and unconscious, it is concerned with the poetic faculty. Giving shape to life, secondary imagination dissolves and reintegrates components to create new meaning (http://romantic-poets.bloomy-ebooks.com/2014/12/coleridges-distinction-between-primary.html).
6 Sefirot are symbols through which the Kabbalists attempted to apprehend the nature of God. They may also be thought of as archetypes of values and ways of being (Drob, 2000; Starr, 2008).
7 The Kabbalists maintain that the letters in a name embody the essence of the thing itself. From "nothing" comes "I" or will (desire), the first named sefirot. *Ayin* (nothing) and *Ani* (I) contain the same Hebrew consonants (*aleph*, *yud*, *nun* or AYN), implying that "nothing" undergoes a change to become the eternal "I" or Divine will. Being and nothingness are always present in creation. Nothingness must be crossed over for transformation to occur (Drob, 2000).
8 Meant as tools to reflect on the psychoanalytic process, the terms alpha and beta refer to how to turn unmetabolized or raw bits of emotional experience (beta elements) into usable thoughts (alpha elements). The alpha function in the analyst works on the patient's undigested thoughts, feelings and sensations and makes them available to the patient so meaning can be created (Bion, 1962). Beta elements, on the other hand, manifest in projective identifications and contribute to acting out.
9 The Midrash Tanchuma is a collection of stories, discussions of specific laws and rabbinical offerings all connected to the Torah, helping to make the, at times, terse language of the bible more accessible (https://www.sefaria.org/Midrash_Tanchuma%2C_Introduction?lang=bi).

References

Aron, L. (2005). The tree of knowledge: Good and evil conflicting interpretations. *Psychoanalytic Dialogues*, 15:681–707.
Balint, M. (1968). *The basic fault*. London: Tavistock.

Bion, W.R. (1962). *Learning from experience.* London: Heinemann.
Bion, W.R. (1967). *Second thoughts: Selected papers on psycho-analysis.* London: Heinemann.
Bion, W.R. (1977). *Seven servants: Four works by Bion.* ,Northvale, NJ: Jason Aronson.
Bion, W.R. (1988). Notes on memory and desire. In E.B. Spillius (Ed.), *Melanie Klein today: Developments in theory and practice, Vol. 2. Mainly practice* (pp. 15–18). New York: Routledge.
Bromberg, P.M. (2013). Hidden in plain sight: Thoughts on imagination and the lived unconscious. *Psychoanalytic Dialogues*, 23:1–14.
Buber, M. (1970). *I and thou. A new translation, with a prologue and notes by Walter Kaufmann.* New York: Touchstone.
Buber, M. (1991). *Tales of the Hasidim.* (O. Marx, Trans.). New York: Schocken Books.
Csikszentmihalyi, M. (1990). *Flow: The psychology of optimal experience.* New York: Harper & Row.
Csikszentmihalyi, M. (1996). *Creativity: Flow and the psychology of discovery and invention.* New York: Harper Collins.
Domash, L. (2009). The emergence of hope: Implicit spirituality in treatment and the occurrence of "psychoanalytic luck." *Psychoanalytic Review*, 96:35–54.
Domash, L. & Shapiro, R.P. (April 19, 2012). Psychoanalyst/mother and artist/daughter dialogue about flow and creativity in art and psychoanalysis. 32nd Annual Spring Meeting of the Division of Psychoanalysis (39) of the American Psychological Association, *The Leading Edge of Creativity*, Santa Fe, NM.
Domash, L. (2014a). Creating "therapeutic" space: How architecture and design can inform psychoanalysis. *Psychoanalytic Perspectives*, 11:94–111.
Domash, L. (2014b). Intergenerational dreaming: Response to Gerald and Sperber. *Psychoanalytic Perspectives*, 11:133–137.
Drob, S.L. (2000). *Kabbalistic metaphors: Jewish mystical themes in ancient and modern thought.* Northvale, NJ: Jason Aronson.
Eigen, M. (1981). The area of faith in Winnicott, Lacan and Bion. *International Journal of Psycho-Analysis*, 62:413–433.
Fromm, E. (1966). *You shall be as gods: A radical interpretation of the Old Testament and its tradition.* New York: Holt, Rinehart and Winston.
Gerald, M. (2011). The psychoanalytic office: Past, present and future. *Psychoanalytic Psychology*, 28(3):435–445.
Ghent, E. (1990). Masochism, submission, surrender – Masochism as a perversion of surrender. *Contemporary Psychoanalysis*, 26:108–136.
Gordon, K. (2004). The Tiger's Stripe: Some thoughts on psychoanalysis, gnosis and the experience of wonderment. *Contemporary Psychoanalysis*, 40:5–45.
Green, A. (1999). *The work of the negative.* London: Free Association Books.
Griffiths, R.R., Johnson, M.W., Richards, W.A., Richards, B.D., McCann, U.D. & Jesse, R. (2011). Psilocybin occasioned mystical-type experiences: Immediate and persisting dose-related effects. *Psychopharmacology (Berl)*, 218(4):649–665.
Griffiths, R.R., Johnson, M.W., Carducci, M.A., Umbricht, A., Richards, W.A., Richards, B.D., Cosimano, M.P. & Klinedinst, M.A. (2016). Psilocybin produces substantial and sustained decrease in depression and anxiety in patients with

life-threatening cancer: A randomized double-blind trial. *Journal of Psychopharmacology*, 30(12):1181–1197.
Griffiths, R.R., Richards, W.A., Johnson, M.W., McCann, U.D. & Jesse, R. (2008). Mystical-type experiences occasioned by psilocybin mediate the attribution of personal meaning and spiritual significance 14 months later. *Journal of Psychopharmacology*, 22(6):621–632.
Grossmark, R. (2012). The unobtrusive relational analyst. *Psychoanalytic Dialogues*, 22:629–646.
Herreman, F. (2002). *Facing the mask*. New York: Museum for African Art.
Hillman, J. (1992). *Re-visioning psychology*. New York: Harper Perennial.
Hoffman, M. (2011). *Towards mutual recognition: Relational psychoanalysis and the Christian narrative*. New York: Routledge.
Lehrer, J. (July 28, 2008). The Eureka Hunt. *The New Yorker*, 40–45.
Limb, C.J. & Braun, A.R. (2008). Neural substrates of spontaneous musical performance: An fMRI study of jazz improvisation. *PLoS ONE*, 3(2):e1679. https://doi.org/10.1371/journal.pone.0001679
MacLean, K.A., Johnson, M.W. & Griffiths, R.R. (2011). Mystical experiences occasioned by the hallucinogen psilocybin lead to increases in the personality domain of openness. *Journal of Psychopharmacology*, 25(11):1453–1461.
Ogden, T.H. (1989). *The primitive edge of experience*. Northvale, NJ: Jason Aronson.
Ogden, T.H. (1994). The analytic third: Working with intersubjective clinical facts. *International Journal of Psycho-Analysis*, 75:3–19.
Ogden, T.H. (2004). This art of psychoanalysis: Dreaming undreamt dreams and interrupted cries. *International Journal of Psycho-Analysis*, 85:857–877.
Ogilvie, J. (April 2002). On emptiness, language and the psychoanalytic self. Paper presented at the 22nd annual meeting of the Division of Psychoanalysis (39), New York, NY.
Ross, S., Bossis, A., Guss, J., Agin-Liebes, G., Malone, T., Cohen, B., Mennenga, S.E., Belser, A., Kalliontzi, K., Babb, J., Su, Z., Corby, P. & Schmidt, B.L. (2016). Rapid and sustained symptom reduction following psilocybin treatment for anxiety and depression in patients with life-threatening cancer: A randomized controlled trial. *Journal of Psychopharmacology*, 30(12):1–16.
Sayers, J. (2002). Mysticism and psychoanalysis: The case of Marion Milner. *International Journal of Psycho-Analysis*, 83:105–120.
Schwartz, H. (2007). *Tree of souls: The mythology of Judaism*. New York: Oxford Universities Press.
Soloveitchik, J.B. (1983). *Halakhic man*. Philadelphia, PA: Jewish Publication Society.
Starr, K. (2008). *Repair of the soul: Metaphors of transformation in Jewish mysticism and psychoanalysis*. New York: Routledge.
Stern, D.N., Sander, L., Nathan, J., Harrison, A., Bruschweiler-Stern, N. & Tronick, E. (1998). Non-interpretive mechanisms in psychoanalytic therapy: The 'something more' than interpretation. *International Journal of Psycho-Analysis*, 79:903–921.
Tagliazucchi, E., Carhart-Harris, R., Leech, R., Nutt, D. & Chialvo, D.R. (2014). Enhanced repertoire of brain dynamical states during the psychedelic experience. *Human Brain Mapping*, 35:5442–5456.

Talamo, P.B. (2018). *Maps for psychoanalytic exploration*. New York: Routledge.
Winkler, G. & Elior, L.B. (1994). *The place where you are standing is holy: A Jewish theology on human relationships*. Northvale, NJ: Jason Aronson.
Winnicott, D.W. (Ed.) (1965). The capacity to be alone. In *The maturational processes and the facilitating environment* (pp. 29–36). London: Karnac.
Winnicott, D.W. (Ed.) (1975). Metapsychological and clinical aspects of regression within the psycho-analytical set-up. In *Through paediatrics to psycho-analysis* (pp. 278–294). New York: Basic Books.
Winnicott, D.W. (1971). *Playing and reality*. London: Tavistock.
Woodman, M. (2011). Coming to a door. In S. Aizenstat & R. Bosnak (Eds.), *Imagination in medicine* (pp. xi–xiv). New Orleans, LA: Spring Journal Books.
Zornberg, A. (2015). Bewilderments: The story of the spies. In L. Aron & L. Henik (Eds.), *Answering a question with a question: Contemporary psychoanalysis and Jewish thought Volume 11* (pp. 99–132). Brighton, MA: Academic Studies Press.
Zornberg, A. & Tippet, K. (October 6, 2011). The genesis of desire. Interview by K. Tippet, *On Being*.

Chapter 3

Unconscious communication and the uncanny

> 'There's no use trying,' [Alice] said: 'one *can't* believe impossible things.'
> 'I daresay you haven't had much practice,' said the Queen. 'When I was your age, I always did it for half-an-hour a day. Why, sometimes I've believed as many as six impossible things before breakfast.'
> (Carroll, 1872/2015, p. 208)

The psychoanalyst Paula Hamm made it a habit to sit quietly for a period of time during the course of a week. Relaxing, with her eyes closed, she suddenly saw an image of a young boy putting a plastic bag over his head. Very disturbed, she had no idea who the boy was. Then a few hours later, a patient came in very upset, telling her his young son had put a plastic bag over his head over the weekend (Mayer, 2007).

I had a similar experience. Right before a patient entered my office for a session, I was opening the window and several phrases floated into my mind, "falling down the rabbit hole" and her "goose was cooked" – maybe drifting into my *Alice in Wonderland* mode. Then, as soon as the session started, the patient immediately used these phrases, although I never remembered her (or me) using them before. Was I reading her mind or was she reading mine?

Listening to a series of her patient's dreams, Melanie Suchet (2004) describes how she became aware that her patient had uncanny knowledge of intimate details of Suchet's life, including her decision to become pregnant and then, very early on, of her actual pregnancy. She and her patient were having a mutual unconscious dialogue, although her patient was unaware of this.

Where do these thoughts come from? Maybe they are pure coincidence or maybe information conveyed in a previous session. Had I ever mentioned my fascination with *Alice in Wonderland* to my patient? Or could these be instances of mind-to-mind communication without external clues?

As we travel in the patient's imaginative world – the dizzying, provocative land of waking and sleeping dreams – we do, at times, seem to read minds. The patient, of course, walks in our world as well. This play and interplay are the stuff of discovery and creation. In this chapter, I shall explore various iterations of the relational/resonant imagination, which can seem uncanny. Therapists experience nonverbal communication (tone/prosody of voice, bodily movements, gestures) unconsciously, mainly body to body, such as when Steven Knoblauch (2005) turns his clinical attention to the shifts of movement and sound in his patient's body as they resonate with his own. Other times thoughts pass between patient and therapist in session by less obvious means or even at a distance, such as when patient or therapist becomes aware of something about the other when not in each other's presence.

In all of these instances, there is deep resonance between the therapist and patient. In an interesting study, Alejandro Pérez et al. (2017) report that the rhythms of brainwaves between two people in conversation begin to match each other. This interbrain synchrony may be a key factor in interpersonal communication. Analogously, scientists report that two pendulum clocks set at different times against a wall side by side eventually beat in unison. As pendulums move back and forth, sound pulses travel through the wall from clock to clock. These pulses can interfere with the swings of the pendulums, eventually causing them to synchronize (Oliveira & Melo, 2015).

Unconscious communications or seemingly telepathic phenomena have been reported by writers (Balint, 1955; Schmeidler, 1966; Ehrenwald, 1978; Marks-Tarlow, 2020 among others)[1] who have suggested they represent either side of the clinical dyad attempting to break through resistance to reach the other. This resonates. At times when patients seem trapped in secondary process or very logical, rational thinking, I employ a form of paranormal phenomena or psi[2] to get a sense of what's going on "underneath." I try to forget logic, toss off judgment, know "nothing" and become a blank slate on which my unconscious can write. I assume a meditative stance and pay close attention to whatever mental image appears to me, which may or may not be related. I am reminded of an artist, Leelee Kimmel, who said, "My paintings are only good when I'm not aware of what I'm doing..." (Duray, 2018, p. 3).

In these instances, when the thought or image wells up in me, it almost feels like it is coming from the outside, like the voice is being *sent* to me but yet is *within* me. Maybe this is what Yeats meant when he talked about his "automatic writing," when the writer suspends his conscious mind and lets his hand move across the paper, seemingly directed by outside forces and/or the unconscious. My experience of "hearing" this type of internal voice is interesting but eerie. Could I be "hearing" the unspoken voice of the patient? Is something formerly invisible now visible? Is my right brain (imagistic, nonlinear, wholistic thinking) talking to my left brain (linguistic, logical, specific thinking)?[3] The experience does seem close to magic.

After the image bubbles up, I may use it in some way with the patient, either translated into alpha, to borrow Bion's term, or occasionally, utter it raw. For example, a retired accountant, my patient was very much staying on the surface with the "facts," as he told me about a new woman he was dating. I felt constrained by his literal account. I let my mind go and had an image of a red checked gingham apron. I said that to him, and he startled. Then he paused for a moment and said that his frequently depressed mother wore a gingham apron when she was making dinner. He usually feels very little sense of connection to her and denies a sense of loss at their lack of connection. However, the mention of the apron startled him, and he had a memory of longing. He sensed how he would come into the kitchen, wanting to connect and feeling despondent at her lack of attention to him. This helped us reach an undercurrent of emotional vitality in him, which had been missing. Again, this could be mere coincidence, or my association to the style of the era of his childhood, but it did unlock a suppressed area of emotion. My imaginative musing, which included the suspension of logical and critical thinking, led him to grasp more deeply his complicated relationship with his mother rather than his usual literal understanding of events.

Of note, Milner (2010) in *On Not Being Able to Paint* writes about this aspect of the creative process. Whenever something new emerged in her painting, Milner experienced a surrender, a blanking out of ordinary consciousness. Her usual sense of self seemed to temporarily disappear. Composers, for example, often experience a surrender of their usual consciousness to a musical idea, which seems to comes from an external source. Mozart said he was not a composer, merely God's assistant in creation. Milner goes on to ask if this may not also reflect an essential part of the creative process, not just of art but also of living. These are "moments in which there is a plunge into no-differentiation which results (if all goes well) in a reemerging into a new division of the me-not-me …?" (Milner, 2010, p. 181), that is, a new creation.

As has been discussed from a neuroscience point of view, the suspension of self-monitoring and self-censoring processes is necessary for creativity to proceed (Limb & Braun, 2008). This suspension may aid unconscious communication and the activation of the relational imagination. Limb and Braun posit that deactivating the center in the brain, the dorsolateral prefrontal cortex (DLPFC), that self-censors may be associated with the kind of free-floating attention that permits spontaneous unplanned associations and sudden insights or realizations. These may be moments, to use Ghent's term, of "surrender," similar to Milner's descriptions of the blanking out of ordinary consciousness that allows something new to emerge.

The issue of therapeutic attunement, as in the moment of my seeing the image of the red-checked gingham apron, is particularly meaningful as intuitive attunement to the patient may be more critical in bringing about psychological change than particular techniques or interpretations (Schore, 2006). Evidence-based practice research also leads to the conclusion that the quality of the bond between patient and therapist plays a larger role in positive change in psychotherapy than does any specific technical or theoretical approach (Horvath, 2001; Lambert & Barley, 2001; Ardito & Rabellino, 2011).

There may be a resurgence of interest in extraordinary perception or psi with the advent of relational school of psychoanalysis with its disavowal of neutrality and interest in attunement and unconscious communication, especially the mutual influence of the therapist/analyst and patient on each other. In this context, the clinician's subjectivity is cultivated as a primary tool of knowledge. She must continuously and imaginatively work to enter the meditative flow of the session, remain open to positive and negative unconscious thoughts and venture into potential emptiness with the faith it will eventually yield good results.

This type of attention encourages the exploration of psi. In fact, Susan Lazar (2001) asks us to consider our relationship with the patient in the context of the possibility of paranormal phenomena. For example, what influences might the therapist's reverie have on the patient's free associations? We may have to rethink the power of our negative and positive intentions toward our patients and theirs toward us, *even* when we are not in their presence.

Fear of psi

Psi phenomena can be frightening, and we may tend to avoid or deny them. Freud's discussion of the uncanny helps us understand our fear (Freud, 1919). He refers to *heimlich*, German for familiar, or another meaning, that which is hidden and should remain secret. When *heimlich* is revealed, it becomes *unheimlich*, meaning frightening and uncanny. Freud refers to Friedrich Schelling's definition of the uncanny "as something which ought to have remained hidden but has come to light" (1919, p. 224). This happens in psi phenomena: a telepathic experience, what was invisible, that is, existed only in the other person's mind, becomes visible to the telepathic individual and creates an eerie feeling.

This also happens in the creative act – something comes into consciousness we may have tried to hide, perhaps an activation of a traumatic memory. The invisible becomes visible, in the process of psychotherapy or between the artist and her art. This can arouse dread and fear. To work frightening feelings through in the act of creation, we need to let down defensive barriers (Ghent, 1990), including giving up familiar ways of seeing, that is, recontextualize memory, to allow something new to appear. The act of surrender helps us be in the moment in order to "find" our creation, something unique and our own. Surrender, in this sense, facilitates growth and liberation.

Many clinicians express interest and/or belief in psi in private but are fearful of the consequences if their ideas become public (Farrell, 1983; Mayer, 2001, 2007). An example is Robert Stoller's 1973 unpublished paper on telepathy, which was published posthumously by Elizabeth Lloyd Mayer (2001). Stoller relates a series of telepathic dreams, his own and his patients, mainly with the goal of "responsible data collecting concerning apparently anomalous, possibly telepathic experiences" (Mayer, 2001, p. 631). These are dreams in which the dreamer is aware of a fact in the world before actually being told about it.

One example is Stoller's dream about Ralph Greenson's son when Stoller was in supervision with Greenson. Greenson's son, a medical student, had been in a motorcycle accident over the weekend, in which he was almost killed. Shortly after this happened, Stoller arrived for supervision and, for the first time instead of just saying "hello," he asked Greenson how he was. Greenson explained the terrible experience over the weekend when his son had an accident, resulting a compound fracture of the left leg. Stoller was astonished, as he had dreamt over the weekend of a medical student being brought into the emergency room with a compound fracture of the left leg due to a motorcycle accident. According to Greenson's son, whom Mayer contacted for her article, Greenson was both disturbed and impressed by Stoller's dream. Despite holding to a strict scientific standard and opposed to anything considered mystical, Greenson felt that Stoller's dream was inexplicably telepathic. However, for the sake of Stoller's reputation, Greenson advised against publishing it.

"Psi shock" in therapy

The following demonstrates of how an analyst's telepathically uttered remark closed a communication gap between herself and her patient, a phenomenon discussed earlier. After Ruth Rosenbaum (2011) spontaneously uttered a seemingly telepathic communication, she reports how the patient felt more understood and the intersubjective field shifted.

As background, Rosenbaum's patient Carla feared her mother was trying to poison her, including via the telephone or by giving her completely inappropriate gifts. Carla felt she had to accept these gifts, even though each time she would fall into a deep depression. Rosenbaum was dreading Carla's upcoming birthday, as she knew her mother would send another "gift." After her birthday, Carla came to session and started to explain how she slowly began to open her mother's gift. Then before Carla could describe the actual gift, Rosenbaum (2011, p. 83) blurted out, "Oh, no! Mustard and fuchsia plaid! That's awful!" In her mind's eye, Rosenbaum saw the article of clothing.

The patient was shocked, exclaiming, "How did you know? It was a mustard and purple plaid jumper. A jumper! Who wears jumpers? And those colors! So ugly – how did you know?"

Mortified, Rosenbaum felt her analyzing instrument has gone haywire. She was afraid Carla would again feel poisoned. However, Carla was relieved. She felt that now Rosenbaum knew how she feels. In fact, the patient jokingly said that now the analyst had her disease too! Playing along, Rosenbaum said they had to find an "antidote" before Easter, as neither of them could take another poisoning. From here on, Carla seemed more open to interpretations. When the Easter gift came from her mother, Carla was able to throw it away without opening it.

How might we understand what occurred with Carla? Rosenbaum speculates that Carla's unconscious need for an attuned mother was so compelling that it provoked Rosenbaum's unconscious to produce the psi event, thereby creating an experience of early mother-infant attunement, an example of the relational imagination. Rosenbaum turns to Theodor Reik (1972, pp. 139–140) for an explanation. He describes ways of sensing that at times may bypass or override normal sensory routes, "Possibly these unknown senses work faster than those we know, can communicate their perceptions to the unconscious faster than the senses developed later, and so seem to act through the air." More recently, Ofra Eshel (2006, p. 1622) writes about "patient-analyst unconscious interconnectedness and its 'impossible' extremes, defying space, time and personal boundaries."

This intense need of Carla for an attuned mother is similar to the intense need an artist has to create and produce works from his imagination. An example close to home, I *need* to write this book, working for hours and hours, out of a strong need to clarify, master and produce material but mostly to create something that is *attuned* to my inner being. The book slowly became a symbiotic object, with which I feel close yet, at times, despise. It is so hard to bring it into being (you could say so hard to find the true self) yet I am totally devoted to it and need to see it through to the end. Perhaps as Christopher Bollas (2011) writes, I am in search of a transformational object. Although I have gotten much help from mentors and friends, as a writer I have to create the object primarily by myself whereas in the above example, Carla had Dr. Rosenbaum. I would also venture that I hope that we – you as reader and I as author – will be attuned to, and learn from, each other.

Even Freud dabbled in the occult

Instructing the analyst "to catch the drift of the patient's unconscious with his own unconscious," Freud (1923, p. 239) was the first to suggest our own unconscious as an analyzing instrument, including the passing of thoughts between the mind of the analyst and patient without visible means. In Freud's words, the analyst "... must turn his own unconscious like a receptive organ towards the transmitting unconscious of the patient. He must adjust himself to the patient as a telephone receiver is adjusted to the transmitting microphone" (Freud, 1912, pp. 115–116). Several years later he writes, "It is a very remarkable thing that the unconscious of one human being can react upon that of another, without passing through the conscious. This deserves closer investigation ... but, descriptively speaking, the fact is incontestable" (1915, p. 194).

Continuing to explore the unconscious transfer of thoughts and feelings, Freud (1921, 1922, 1925, 1933, 1941) wrote "mental processes in one person – ideas, emotional states, conative impulses – can be transferred to another person through empty space without employing the familiar methods of communication by means of words and signs" (Freud, 1933, p. 39). He continued that:

> The telepathic process is supposed to consist in a mental act in one person instigating the same mental act in another person. What lies between these two mental acts may easily be a physical process into which the mental one is transformed at one end and which is transformed back once more into the same mental one at the other end.
>
> (Freud, 1933, p. 55)

For Freud, telepathy was an activity of the unconscious mind, and just as with dreams, much can be learned about unconscious feelings from telepathically (unconsciously) received material. Broadly speaking, what Freud referred to as telepathy, we think of as unconscious communication.

Observing fortune tellers, Freud (1921) illustrated how an unconscious wish, along with the thoughts and factual material connected with it, could be transferred from one person to another. In Freud's view, some of the fortune tellers' errors came from understanding their clients' inner psychic reality (unspoken wishes and fantasies) better than their external reality. In this sense, the occult benefits from psychoanalytic understanding, which helps make sense of the fortune teller's prophecies, which may be more metaphorically than actually true.

He cites one case in which the fortune teller told the client that his brother-in-law, a hated rival, would die from crayfish poisoning in August. (The only information the client had given the fortune teller was the brother-in-law's birthdate, without even telling her who the person was.) The brother–in-law did not die but did, in fact, have intense crayfish poisoning in August and almost died. The fortune teller, according to Freud's reasoning, telepathically sensed the intensely destructive wishes of the client toward his brother-in-law so strongly, a phenomenon Freud (1921, p. 184) referred to as "thought transference,"[4] that the fortune teller interpreted this to mean the brother-in-law would die.

Almost a hundred years later, current discussion of mirror neurons, emotional resonance and fractal theory, all discussed later in this chapter, support Freud's strong hunch that thought transference would be accepted as scientific fact. However, despite his convictions, Freud was very circumspect in his discussion of psychic phenomena. While Freud remarked to an acquaintance Hereward Carrington, a British psychical researcher, that if he had his life to live over again, he would rather study psychical phenomena than psychoanalysis, he subsequently "forgot" he said this. Ernest Jones, however, found the letter to Carrington, which confirmed the statement (Jones, 1957). Another example is Freud's remark to Jones, who criticized Freud's interest in clairvoyance, "I don't like it at all myself, but there is some truth in it" (Jones, 1957, p. 381).

In his correspondence with Sandor Ferenczi, Freud highlighted his ambivalence. Over a period of many years, Freud encouraged and participated in Ferenczi's experiments with thought transference but also expressed anxiety about expressing these ideas publicly (Brabant et al., 1993; Falzeder & Brabant, 1996). In a letter to Ferenczi in December, 1910, Freud wrote:

> I see destiny approaching, inexorably, and I note that it has designated you to bring to light mysticism and the like. ... Still, I think we ought to venture to slow it down. I would like to request that you continue to research in secrecy for two full years and don't come out until 1913 – you know my practical reasons against it and my secret painful sensitivities.
> (Brabant et al., 1993, p. 240)

Of note, Carl Jung (1989) speculated that Freud's emphasis on repressed sexuality was, in part, a means of repressing something even more disturbing to Freud's notion of adult consciousness: mysticism.

Despite reservations, Freud continued to pursue the subject. By 1933, when he published Dreams and Occultism, he enthusiastically delves into an investigation of occult phenomena, for the most part using the same examples as in his 1921 paper while adding a case. In this additional case, Freud gives the account of a mother who spoke during her analytic session of a gold coin important to her in childhood. Uncannily, as soon as she arrived home from the session, her ten-year-old son came to her with a gold coin to keep for him. He had gotten it months ago, so there was no particular reason why on that day he would remember the gold coin. A few weeks later, the mother was sitting at her desk to write about this coincidence. Eerily, at that moment, the boy who was also in analysis came in and asked for the gold coin back to show it to his analyst (Freud, 1933).

Freud speculated that in the course of evolution, telepathy, a more primal, archaic form of communication, has been replaced by giving signals, such as speech, which are picked up by sense organs. However, the older method may remain and function under certain conditions, such as in psychoanalysis. Freud also speculated that this might be the form of communication in insect communities that develop a common sense of purpose (Freud, 1933). This type of primal communication is seen between mother and infant, as each communicates with the other without words, through deep intuition. The good mother imaginatively picks up many subliminal cues that guide her in responding to her child.

Ferenczi, the "thought reader"

In contrast to the ambivalence of Freud, Ferenczi wholly believed in the occult and referred to himself as a wonderful "thought-reader" (cited in Stanton, 1990, p. 89). He explained that through his own free associations, he could imaginatively read the thoughts of his patients. Patients were also able to perceive his unconscious psychic experiences, as in the example of Suchet's patient described earlier. Ferenczi referred to the "dialogues of unconsciouses" (Bass, 2001, p. 687) in which "the unconsciousness of two people completely understand themselves and each other, without the remotest conception of this on the part of the consciousness of either" (Ferenczi, 1980, p. 109; see also Hidas, 1993).

From the start of their relationship in 1908, Ferenczi wanted this kind of close, mind-to-mind relationship with Freud. Ferenczi yearned for "mutual openness ... useful, clear-as-day openness, which conceals nothing" and thought this was possible between two psychoanalytically minded people such as Freud and himself (Brabant et al., 1993, October 3, 1910, quoted in Aron, 1998, p. 9). Freud, however, rejected his entreaties for complicated theoretical and personal reasons (Aron, 1998).

Later in 1926, concerned about Freud's mental and physical health, which Ferenczi likely saw as interconnected, Ferenczi offered to travel to Vienna to analyze Freud. Freud had been diagnosed with cancer of the jaw three years earlier and was now also suffering with heart problems (Falzeder et al., 2000). Robert Kramer (2003) suggests that Ferenczi might very well have felt that Freud's oral cancer was a kind of "teratoma," Ferenczi's term for a physical expression of isolated fragments of infantile experience and emotions, the return, so to speak, of the repressed. Freud graciously rejected Ferenczi's offer, although he did acknowledge there could be a psychological aspect to his physical condition.

Ferenczi's openness to a mystical exchange can be understood in a cultural context as well. In the intellectual life of Vienna at the turn of the century, there was a diffuse sense that the boundary between the ego and the world is permeable, that all is in flux. There was strong interest in the occult, which was in conflict with the development of 20th century science, to which Freud was wedded, both by his training and his wish to have psychoanalysis accepted.

Fast forward to current thinking

Symbiotic phenomena or boundary blurring in psychotherapy

Psi phenomena and transitional space can be thought of as parallel phenomena. In the transitional area of blurred boundaries and intense experiencing, symbiotic phenomena are more likely to occur. The therapist's analyzing instrument, which allows for unconscious understanding of the patient's communications based in part on the therapist's shift toward primary process thinking, may be viewed as an example of transitional or symbiotic phenomena (Balter et al., 1980; Rosenbaum, 2011).[5] As Leon Balter et al.

(1980, p. 474) note, the analyzing instrument is not a separate entity within the clinician but a joint construction of the therapeutic dyad "functioning together as one unit in continuous communication." An interplay of primary and secondary processes (see endnote 5), this is a creative act by the clinician and her patient.

Boundary blurring moments between patient and therapist may be necessary for deep change to occur. As Harold Searles (1976) and others have written, during this process, the therapist introjects the patient's conflicts and, with his relatively strong ego, deals with these both consciously and unconsciously. Then the patient by introjection benefits from this intrapsychic therapeutic work. Similarly, Gaetano Benedetti (1987) writes, "the birth of the self is composed of a mixture of interchangeable parts of oneself and others" (p. 194).

Related, Bollas (2011) writes that we underestimate the adult's search for a transformational object,[6] which will provide experiences reminiscent of the early infant/mother symbiosis, where we feel a oneness and an opportunity for transcendence. As we experience our deficits, we long for union with a presence that will metamorphize the self. Indeed, according to Kabbalah, even God needs a transformational object. His intense longing to be affirmed by the human being is seen as the motivation for creation (Starr, 2008). God desires that we desire him and enter into relationship with him (Zornberg & Tippet, 2011). Lawrence Kushner, noted biblical scholar, explains that Kabbalah attains maturity as "a system of theosophy, claiming to explain the influence of human action on the inner life of God" (Kushner & Tippet, 2014).

God grows to know himself through his interactions with man. As the Kabbalist Chayyim Vital (quoted in Drob, 2000, p. 25) phrased it, "if there was no one in the world who could receive (God's) mercy how could He be called merciful?" Also, by God's allowing for the possibility of evil in the world, humankind is faced with the necessity of making choices that fully actualize the values (the sefirot discussed in Chapter 2) that lie at the core of God (Drob, 2000). Through this repair of the world, we complete and transform God and ourselves.

God's longing to be known is referred to as God's "crisis" (Scholem, 1995). This is what motivates God to go from hidden to revealed, from repose to activity, passing through no-thing, as He creates the world. As Starr writes, no-thingness is liminal space, a "stage of reality that lies between being wholly within the One and the first glimpse of a separate existence" (Green, 2004, p. 38 quoted in Starr, 2008, p. 72). This parallels the concept of transitional space, defined by Winnicott as movement from the purely subjective world of union with the mother to the gradual entry into the objectivity of separateness (Winnicott, 1971).

This moment between *oneness* and *being* is named by the Kabbalist Azreil of Gerona as a point of faith (Drob, 2000). Patient and therapist must have the faith to go into this in-between space and, at times, tolerate shattering, just as the vessels shattered when God created the world. The therapeutic dyad needs faith to tolerate the formlessness, chaos and anxiety that may precede the reorganization and creation of a truer self.

Kabbalah empathizes that the world is in continuous creation. There is no such thing as time for God. The past, present and future are continuous reality, and the world's coming into being is continuous. When we are close to God and have faith, we feel the same way. The divine is always present, and it is always possible to repair the world (Kushner & Tippet, 2014). This translates to psychotherapy. Our patients pass through the space of no-thing, the transitional arena on the way to wholeness. In this space, the boundaries between the patient and therapist lessen, as each loosens rigidities and surrenders to the process, much as the Kabbalists describe a mystical moment with God. In these moments we know new creations of the self are possible, that we – both therapist and patient – have within us the possibility of ongoing repair and rebirth. For the Kabbalists and, hopefully, for the therapeutic dyad, the coming into being is continuous. *Creation is now.*

Magical thinking

Part of psychoanalysis' long antipathy to anything that feels nonscientific or cannot be proven is an unwillingness to acknowledge the role played by magical thinking in the analytic encounter. Belief in psi may be viewed as a form of magical thinking, which can be defined as "the belief that thoughts and desires can directly transfer themselves to, and transform, the material world, other people, the future" (Thurschwell, 2005, p. 6).

According to some anthropologists, magical thinking is considered the most primitive mode of thought. As evolution progresses, magical thinking is followed by religious thinking and finally by scientific and analytical thinking (Frazer, 1994; Pacini & Epstein, 1999; Mauss, 2001).[7] Indirect support for this comes from research indicating that people with paranormal beliefs are somewhat less likely to think critically (Epstein et al., 1996; Pacini & Epstein, 1999; Brottman, 2009). However, we all have many different modes of processing information, which, broadly speaking, may be divided into two kinds: the intuitive and the analytic, each relying on different areas in the brain with different rules of operation (Sloman, 1996; Stanovich & West, 2000; Evans, 2003; Sun et al., 2005; Brottman, 2009). Critical thinking does not replace intuition as the mind matures; rather, as cognitive psychologist Jonathan Evans (2003) suggests, both types of thinking continue to exist and develop throughout life. As we learn more about the scientific basis for Freud's thought transference, the somewhat pejorative term "magical thinking" may become outmoded.

There is the suggestion that beginning in childhood, magical thinking and imagination enrich and enhance each other, and that this continues throughout life (Rosengren & French, 2015). Magical thinking remains operative in dreams and may play a central role in the arts (Subbotsky, 2010).

The idea that magical thinking fosters creativity was tested experimentally by Eugene Subbotsky (2010). He showed one group of children clips from movies depicting magical ideas and another group clips with nonmagical themes from the same movies to determine if after viewing, the first group expressed more creativity. Although additional research is needed, this study suggests that magical thinking does increase creativity, possibly because it facilitates taking into account alternative manifestations of cause and effect and therefore widens perspective. This relates to my implied suggestion that consideration of the *possibility* of psi may stimulate psychotherapeutic creativity.

Is projective identification a form of telepathy?

Projective identification is a particularly fascinating aspect of unconscious communication.[8] In this dynamic, the patient unconsciously and powerfully projects onto the therapist an unwanted or painful part of the self; the therapist feels this is her own experience, sometimes to the point of feeling possessed. This is an unconscious transfer of thoughts and feelings between therapist and patient or mind-to-mind communication, the definition of telepathy – a word more commonly used in Freud's time. As mentioned, unconscious communication is the term likely to be used today.

Although based on Freud's concept of psychological projection (1911, 1912–1913) in which one's unacceptable thoughts and feelings are disavowed and attributed to someone else, projective identification is a step beyond. Ogden (1979) writes that projective identification does not just alter the psychological representation of another person, it actually affects the other's feeling state and self-representation. Similarly, in considering projective identification, R.D. Laing (1969) states that the person does not just project his own feelings onto the other but attempts to use the other to embody or feel the projections as if they were his own.

I had a recent experience of projective identification when my six-year-old inhibited patient Lucy was repressing fear and hatred of her mother. She created many drawings in sessions, and in a singsong way, related fairy tale narratives about witches with little emotion. I, on the other hand, began to feel a great deal of emotion in the form of intense persecutory anxiety about her mother, that in some way she would harm me professionally. Feeling helpless in relationship to her mother, I half-consciously experienced her as a scary, evil witch. Needless to say, this was very irrational, except as explained by "thought transference." I was unconsciously absorbing the patient's feelings, which were transferred to me. Only with the help of a colleague was I able to gain perspective and realize that my fear and anxiety was actually my patient's. Her feelings had somehow "flowed" into me. I was then able to experience empathy for my patient, as separate from myself. I was able to more effectively enter her world, especially regarding her drawings, as I deeply "knew" her fear.

I view my terror as a precursor to empathy because, at first, I thought these feelings were my own. I actually thought the mother would hurt me. Empathy as a component of the relational imagination has two parts: first, the therapist experiences the feelings of the patient but then steps back and realizes these are the patient's feelings and not her own. In this case, while the flow of feelings went into me and I experienced them, it only became true empathy when the necessary perspective was taken, and I became aware that these are the patient's feelings.

Exemplifying the underlying metaphoric processes involved in imagination, the act of empathizing utilizes metaphor, as it plays with similarity and difference. The clinician identifies with the patient but at the same time retains her own sense of self. Without this play of similarity/difference, one might experience a total merger with the other. However, with projective identification, the flow of feeling can be so strong that clinicians are in danger of stopping short of the necessary perspective taking.

Conceivably and unfortunately, projective identification could go in the reverse direction as well, with the therapist projecting onto the patient. I recently wrote a farcical comedic play about this. "Two Heads Are Better Than One" takes place during a psychotherapy session and portrays a case of extreme projective identification by the therapist.

The therapist's history included his being sexually overstimulated by his mother, who would sit with him with her breasts exposed. He became obsessed with his mother's breasts and would try to touch them, for which his mother punished him. He projected his obsession onto his patient by linking the patient's depression to her mother's breast cancer. He emphasized this to such an extent that the patient began to be obsessed with her own breasts, convinced that that she had breast cancer, even though she had been told by multiple physicians that she did not. This way the therapist could continuously relive his own trauma of being exposed to, and preoccupied with, his mother's toxic breasts, as the patient constantly discussed her "diseased" breasts with him. The patient also unconsciously colluded in making her breasts "sick" so the therapist would stop short of physically breaking boundaries and actually touch her breasts.

Although this is pure fantasy, it exemplifies the power of projective identification. To create some resolution, the theatrical dialogue in the play utilizes Ferenczi's methods of mutual analysis. The patient eventually suggests they free-associate together, as Ferenczi did with his patients. With this mutual free association, the patient becomes free of the therapist's projections although the therapist remains in an agitated state.

Brief history of the concept

The concept of projective identification has a long history of iterations and reiterations, paralleling the evolution of psychoanalysis itself. Originally viewed in Kleinian terms as a defense, currently it is frequently seen as an attempt to communicate with the analyst. Even the theatrical example of projective identification described above could be viewed as a perverse attempt at communication. The therapist in the play has to rid himself of his disturbing feelings and have someone else (the patient) experience and understand them. The patient then attempts to give them back to him in a digestible fashion.

Referring to unconscious intrapsychic fantasies of the patient, Melanie Klein (1946, 1955) introduced the concept of projective identification in 1946. Klein describes it as a prototype of an aggressive object relationship: the patient has a fantasy of forcibly projecting parts of his disowned self into the analyst, in part, to control the analyst. This can lead to paranoid anxieties as the analyst is then seen as having menacing aspects. The patient can also project a positive aspect of his personality, especially in cases where the patient feels unworthy. Viewing countertransference as an expression of the analyst's pathology, Klein did not explore her countertransference related to the projective identification. Instead, she viewed these feelings as problems to be overcome. However, today post-Kleinians do examine countertransference and see projective identification as an important component of it.

Extending Klein's thinking, Bion (1959) introduced the more dyadic, interactive aspects of projective identification by describing it as a relationship of container and contained. Unlike Klein who saw the projective identification flowing only from patient to analyst, Bion saw the process as a highly interactive, two-mind phenomenon, a communication in which both sides modify the other. Projective identification began to be seen as a valuable source of psychoanalytic information (Rusbridger, 2012) and the creation of something more generative than either participant could create alone.

More recently, Ogden (2004) views projective identification as a particular form of the analytic third, what he terms the subjugating third.[9] For Ogden, analysis is a dialectic between the individual subjectivities of patient and analyst and their cocreated intersubjectivity, the analytic third. In projective identification, the individual subjectivities are temporarily negated. The patient disavows a part of himself and projects this into to the analyst, and the analyst alters himself to receive it. This creates the subjugating third that can experience novel thoughts and feelings, which previously existed only as potential. Both sides unconsciously engage in this to help free the patient, although the analyst too may benefit. If the process is successful, each side of the dyad can then acknowledge the other and reclaim his own identity in order for a new generative dialectic to resume. This is often facilitated by the analyst's interpretations and the patient's ability to respond to them.

Also viewing projective identification as intersubjective, relational thinkers describe this process as a powerful unconscious entreaty by the patient to help put disavowed aspects of the self into words. The projective identification needs to be deeply experienced by another so that it can be worked through (Benjamin, 2004, 2009, 2010; Aron, 2006; Bromberg, 2006; Levine, 2012). However, unlike analysts who advocate these affects be metabolized privately, including Ogden and some post-Kleinians, the relational analyst's experience of projective identification is discussed with the patient at appropriate moments, a continuation of the phenomena termed the "interpersonalization of projective identification" by Mitchell (1995, p. 79). This may help create potential space to process an enactment, a preconscious or unconscious entanglement between patient and therapist. In addition, especially when analysts are open about countertransference, patients can see the analysts' conflicts. As patients probe and question, they may be able to sense how analysts change as a result. When a patient realizes she has been effective in changing her therapist, she may be more able to renegotiate her own conflicts (Slavin & Kriegman, 1998).

Used in a relational context, projective identification allows a patient to look at his own dissociated personality tendencies as the properties of another person, allowing the drama of psychic conflict to be played out interpersonally with the clinician as coparticipant (Blechner, 1994). In order to receive and then explore these projective identifications with the patient, the therapist must have the psychological freedom to consider all sorts of attributions about himself, whether he considers them favorable or unfavorable, plausible or not. He must also, of course, reflect how his experience of projective identification can clarify something about the patient.

The science of unconscious communication and the uncanny

In her groundbreaking discussion of fractals, Terry Marks-Tarlow[10] offers us a way to understand unconscious communication (2008, 2020a,b). Fractal geometry is a relatively new science discovered by Benoit Mandelbrot (1977) in the 1970s. He considered this new branch of mathematics to be the best suited to understand features of the natural world, such as cloud formations and mountain ranges, which had previously been too complicated, ambiguous or irregular to measure. Fractals can also aid in understanding psychological dynamics.

Fractals are nonlinear patterns in nature that continuously evolve. They form infinitely deep patterns upon patterns, multiscaled and recursive – turning back on themselves and beginning again and again. The hallmark of a fractal is a property called self-similarity, which means that the pattern of the whole is reproduced in the pattern of the parts. Think of the branches of a tree. On smaller and smaller scales, the same V shape keeps reappearing over and over. This arc from large scale to small scale pattern is what gives each tree its unique identity.

Psychologically, humans share similar dynamics. Fractal relational patterns are learned early in life. Self-similar patterns build on self-similar patterns, becoming more complex and entrenched with each iteration, creating identity. At various times, different patterns emerge, explaining how different aspects of the self can appear at various moments, depending on the situation (Marks-Tarlow, 1999, 2002, 2004).

In nature, dynamics range from chaotic at one extreme to rigid at the other. The healthiest place tends to be at the edge of chaos, where there is enough chaos to allow novelty but enough rigidity to retain structure. Similar principles hold for human nature, where either extreme – too much chaos or too much rigidity – becomes problematic (Marks-Tarlow, 2008). The repetition compulsion in an individual is an example of a self-similar, rigid fractal pattern. Similarly, intergenerational dysfunctional patterns reverberate in families. Once the patient emotionally recognizes these patterns, they can be easier to change.

Much of the complexity of a fractal lies at its boundaries. Marks-Tarlow (2020a) demonstrates how fractals can model interpenetrating boundaries within highly complex, open systems. Because of their fuzzy, dynamical and flexible nature, fractal boundaries allow for the intermingling of what is inside and what is outside (Marks-Tarlow, personal communication, May 6, 2018). For example, the ocean shoreline with its changing, moment-to-moment shifting delineation has no smooth separation of sand from ocean at water's edge; rather, they interpenetrate each other.

The shoreline can be a metaphor for the psychotherapy process. At points, the ocean (therapist or patient) penetrates high up into the sand (therapist or patient). Other times the ocean moves away, and ocean and sand are more separate. In constant flux, the shoreline is the edge of the process and keeps track. Similarly, boundaries between patient and therapist are dynamic and, at times, fuzzy and flexible. We can seem to interpenetrate each other's minds. This is unconscious communication.

Becoming aware of these patterns or "fractal consciousness" is important for both therapist and patient (Marks-Tarlow, 2008, p. 182). Relating to clinical intuition, fractal consciousness is the capacity to perceive the pattern of the whole from just a thin slice of exposure, or sometimes, in cases of uncanny knowing, from no face-to-face exposure at all. The clinician's ability to identify and understand patterns (within the self and between the self and others) in order to weave together multiple time and event scales into a coherent picture is especially helpful to a patient with a fragmented sense of self. In pointing out how even a small event signifies a larger pattern, the therapist builds structure and provides meaning. The patient's behavior begins to make sense.

The therapist can also point out how a repetitive, dysfunctional (fractal) problem may be reducing in scale. For example, in working with an addict who is despairing that his addictive pattern will always be present, the therapist can explain that while that may be true, the scale of the problem can be gradually reduced so it will not control his life. This reduction in scale becomes evident in the psychotherapy as patient and therapist discuss the dysfunctional patterns on smaller and subtler scales. Whereas initially the patient may have been a frequent binge drinker causing damage to his family and professional life, he is now sober except for very occasional relapses. The relapses can be discussed in therapy and not cause serious disruption in his life.

Turning to a biological understanding, our own physiology is comprised of fractal patterns (Liebovitch, 1998; West, 2016). The neuronal system[11] consists of branching axons and dendrites that spread out in ever-repetitive fractal patterns intersecting with each other. Recent neuroscience research indicates there is very little difference with how one part of our brain communicates with another part (fractal pattern intersecting/interpenetrating with fractal pattern) and how we communicate interpersonally (Kelso et al., 2013). As Marks-Tarlow (2020a, p. 24) writes:

> In other words, how messages are sent from one part of the brain to another share similar coordination dynamics to how messages are sent between brains. Such research points towards fluid, dynamic boundaries between self and other, inner and outer realms.

We intersect with each other – brain-to-brain, mind-to-mind and body-to-body – as we communicate consciously and unconsciously.

Yet we are separate at the same time. J.A. Scott Kelso et al. (2013) report how our fractal brains are in a state of flux, with the elements of synchronization and integration (open, interpenetrating) occurring with elements of segregation and autonomy (closed, separate). The logic of the brain is neither harmony nor separateness but both. Reflecting the activity within our brains, we as therapists are in harmony (synchronization) with our patient while at the same time maintaining our separateness (segregation). This is how we are open and closed at the same time. Take the above example of the red checked gingham apron. In my reverie in transitional space, my boundaries became ever fuzzier and more open. In interaction with my patient, I could somehow "read" his mind while still maintaining my separateness – an example of the relational imagination.

The many fractal neuronal patterns in our brain are part of what makes imagination itself possible. It is the fractal branching pattern of the neuron's axons and dendrites that allows them to communicate with so many other cells. Because of the recurrent branching, our 100 billion neurons can make 100 trillion synaptic connections. That is an average of 1,000 connections per neuron (although some neurons make only one connection and others hundreds of thousands). If instead of fractal patterning, our neurons were shaped like cubes and neatly packed into the brain, one neuron could only connect with, at most, six other cells (Fractal Foundation online course, https://fractalfoundation.org/OFC/OFC-1-1.html). We would have limited ability to create new ideas and structures.

Vittorio Gallese et al. (2007) build on our understanding of unconscious communication through their discovery of mirror neurons.[12] As we observe a person's actions, emotions or physical sensations, the same neural circuits are activated in us as in the person we are observing. Creating a shared body state, this process is unconscious and automatic, and helps us grasp what the other person is thinking and feeling. In other words:

> both therapist and patient may be unconsciously picking up and responding to subtle cues from the other, and the perception of these cues may activate neural patterns shared by both. This process may occur repeatedly in a circular and reciprocal fashion and may constitute the basis for the unconscious communication referred to by Freud.
>
> (Gallese et al., 2007, p. 146)

In a sense, the person performing the action has automatically penetrated the onlooker's brain/mind, like the ocean penetrates the sand. The onlooker then feels what the person performing the action feels, creating a shared body state and reflecting the constant ongoing unconscious communication between people. It is possible that the fractal, fluid nature of our intrabrain and interbrain communication is what makes the synchrony between brains possible. Although at this point highly speculative and in need of further research, it may be that the fractal quality of our nervous system is the bedrock of unconscious communication.

It is interesting that Gallese et al. maintain that mirror neurons cannot account for projective identification, in which the patient's unconscious emotions evoke feelings and thoughts in the analyst *without* any specifically correlated behavioral cues. Mirror neurons only become activated when a movement is involved. Gallese et al. (2007) disagree with the prevailing contemporary psychoanalytic view of the existence and value of projective identification. If there is no neural mechanism involved to account for this phenomenon, then Gallese et al. suggest it is more likely that the analyst's feelings, although perhaps prompted by the patient, arise primarily from circumstances in the analyst's own life and are not a good source of information about the patient.

However, just as we did not understand aspects of the neuroscience of empathy before the discovery of mirror neurons, there may be a future finding that scientifically validates the phenomenon of projective identification (Rosenbaum, 2011). I agree that there is likely a "hook" or vulnerability in the therapist in order to receive the projection but, in my view, we can learn a great deal about the patient if we are able to examine the dissociated affects involved in this phenomenon.

Are psi phenomena scientific?

Will telepathy, a psi phenomenon, be accepted as a scientific fact, as predicted by Freud? Proponents of psi, such as Lazar (2001), Mayer (2007) and Rosenbaum (2011) emphatically state there has been much robust research that is ignored because it does not meet our intuitive sense of how the universe is structured. They stress the need for a revision of our understanding of the physical universe. In his foreword to Mayer's book, *Extraordinary Thinking* (2007), the physicist Freeman Dyson points out that many scientists believe that the results of psi research are disappointing because even when positive, they are still marginal, large enough to be statistically significant but too small to persuade a skeptic. Dyson takes the position that ESP is real but cannot be measured by our current scientific means.

Developments in modern physics make an understanding of psi phenomena easier to conceptualize (Lindley, 1996; Bouwmeester et al., 1997; Radin, 1997 as reported in Lazar, 2001; Suchet, 2016). However, the counterintuitive nature of quantum mechanics, including the fact that nonlocal effects[13] exist and that information can be transmitted instantaneously (Radin, 1997), explains paranormal phenomena *only metaphorically*, not literally.

Bell's theorem, derived mathematically from quantum theory, demonstrated that a pair of particles, once in contact and then moved far apart, would still react simultaneously to stimuli and behave in completely correlated ways. In other words, once-connected particles, even after separation over a great distance, react as if still connected by virtue of an unknown nonlocal effect (Radin, 1997). Albert Einstein called this effect "spooky actions at a distance" (Lindley, 1996).

This prediction has been verified by an experiment which demonstrated that when a pair of previously connected or "entangled" photons are separated, if the first photon acquires a new quantum state such as a new polarization, then the second photon will, even at a distance, also acquire instantaneously the same quantum property (Bouwmeester et al., 1997). Therefore, once two quantum particles intersect, they remain connected and will behave in the same manner, no matter how far apart they are in space and time. According to some interpretations by physicists, this is because they remain as part of a unified waveform, which can extend indefinitely and stretch throughout space. The unified waveform contains the shared information about their quantum states so when one potential particle changes in any way, the other potential particle simultaneously changes as well.

To help us understand this connection regardless of time or space due to an earlier entanglement, the following example is sometimes given. Picture two dice that, when thrown, always register doubles, that is, two threes, two sixes, and so on, no matter how far apart they are. One die could be on earth and the other on Pluto. In the quantum world the waveform for each die entangles and then separates but stays connected. Because of the original entanglement, when one particle changes in some way, the other will also.

Let me give you a clinical example that has metaphorical resonance to the nonlocal effects described by quantum physicists. I was on vacation in Honolulu, Hawaii, nearly 5,000 miles away from my NYC office, when I woke up at 3 AM, very anxious about a patient. When I saw her right after I returned from Hawaii, I learned she was having a violent fight with her mother at that very moment. She told me about how fearful and upset she had been, how she and her mother almost came to physical blows. I was stunned to realize this happened at the same time I woke up and became anxious about her.

In writing about unconscious communication between himself and his patient, Anthony Bass (2001) explores how uncanny connections and the quantum vocabulary of entanglement may reflect the experience of the contemporary psychoanalyst and her patient. He asks if psychoanalysts establish such deep connections with patients that, as with entangled particles, the relationship remains unbroken, no matter how far apart the individuals are in space or time (I hope so!)

Can we think extraordinarily?

Welcome to the puzzling world of psi experiments that involve person-to-person effects at a distance as well as the effects of mind on a machine. I am only able to cite a few select examples, and the interested reader is encouraged to explore the references offered for further, more extensive detail.

Many questions will remain after reading the results of psi experiments below. However, whether or not aspects of psi can be proven scientifically, consideration of these issues expands our imagination and helps us understand our patient more deeply. The information presented is in the spirit of reporting only. It is not meant to vouch for the quality or veracity of the experiments, which is beyond the scope of this chapter (and beyond my ability!).

A series of scientific studies on telepathy have yielded positive results, as reported by Lazar (2001). Two separate meta-analyses of 42 experiments in 34 publications were published in 1985 reporting attempts by the sender to mentally transmit an image to a recipient in a sealed chamber. Of the 28 of the 42 experiments that reported the actual hit rates (as opposed to merely reporting "successful" or "unsuccessful" experiments), the odds against chance of the percentage of accurate perceptions of images "sent" as shown in experiments from ten different labs was ten billion to one. Later studies with better designs replicated these results. This type of study is reminiscent of Rosenbaum's ability to see Carla's plaid jumper in her mind's eye.

Eerie findings about the effect of mind on machine are also reported. One study investigated whether human intention could influence the output of a random event generator's production of 1's or 0's, even when the subject was thousands of miles away. According to chance, the output should be 50% each. A meta-analysis of over 800 experimental studies of the effect of human intention on random event generators, including some conducted by the Princeton Engineering Anomalies Research (PEAR) group,[14] found that human intention could alter the random event generators and that the overall odds against chance of this happening was over a trillion to one (Radin, 1997).

In an interview Rosenbaum conducted with PEAR cofounder Brenda Dunne (interview on February 11, 2004, as cited in Rosenbaum, 2011), Dunne described how some subjects in the experiments attempted to feel merged with the machine, to create a kind of "third space" where they could interact and affect each other. That approach, she said, seemed to produce better results than when subjects tried to exert their will over the machine in a more overt, conscious way. The more successful approach could be described as a kind of meditative state, softening sensations of a separate self and resulting in the experience of a shared space. Bringing to mind Ogden's (1994, 2004) "analytic third," this is analogous to what takes place between therapist and patient in the intersubjective field.

According to Dunne, the word most often used by subjects in the PEAR experiments is "resonate." They tried to resonate with the machine in order to alter the statistically expected patterns. This is similar to our attempts to attune to patients and reach them in a way that might enable them to alter their habitual patterns.

While Mayer (2007) acknowledges psychoanalysis' long-standing skepticism about psi phenomena, her position is that if connectedness rather than separateness moves to the foreground of our awareness, extraordinary knowing is an expectable result of how we view the world. Mayer asks if we as human beings are capable of a connectedness with other people (and every other aspect of our material world) so profound that it breaks all the rules of nature as we know them. For example, in deep meditation, we experience a sense of oneness; there is a literal evaporation of any sense of separation from others or the surrounding world. SPECT studies of monks in deep meditation show a turning down of the posterior superior parietal lobe, a brain area critical to orienting oneself in the physical world. It helps one know his boundaries, where he begins and ends. In deep meditation, as this area is turned down, the sense of these boundaries is removed. Mayer connects this to a feeling of flow and to the type of "knowing" the mystic Buber wrote about. This orientation likely stimulates experience of psi phenomena.

This orientation also facilitates the creative process. As in prayer or meditation, when we create, we are suspended in time, outside of ordinary reality. This suspension of reality, as we usually know it, allows a sense of connection and oneness as well as space for unusual thoughts, new connections and unique perspectives. We effortlessly allow ourselves to come in closer contact with our unconscious, so necessary to create.

Finally, Rosenbaum writes:

> If we take seriously the unconscious communication that occurs in the intersubjective patient-analyst field, and if we accept the research indicating that unconscious mutual influencing is at the core of psychological development from the time we are infants (Beebe & Lachmann, 2002), then psychoanalysts should seriously explore the implications of psi phenomena, where unconscious influencing and communication are the norm. Psi is another royal road, perhaps an expressway, to the unconscious. We should get back on where Freud left off.
>
> (Rosenbaum, 2011, p. 84)

Whether called psi phenomena, transitional experiencing, or the uncanny, these experiences occur in treatment and can help us enter, develop, repair and expand the imagination.

Notes

1 Marks-Tarlow (2020b) gives an example in her patient Sabrina's tidal wave dream, a dream that had the same imagery as Marks-Tarlow's own dreams as a child. Marks-Tarlow and her patient came to view the dream as a transpersonal attempt to create greater empathy in the dyad. As a result of reflecting on the dream, Marks-Tarlow became aware of important countertransference so therapy could proceed.

2 Referring to communication that exceeds common understanding, psi is a term derived from the 23rd letter of the Greek alphabet (psi) and the first letter of the Greek word psyche. Psi encompasses mind-to-mind communication (telepathy); environment-to-mind communication (clairvoyance); and the capacity to influence an object, such as the effect of mind on machine (Rosenbaum, 2011).

3 The difference between the two hemispheres is not so much about what they actually do but in the differing perspectives taken. The left hemisphere is narrower in focus and relatively inflexible. Specialized for speech, it deals more with individual pieces of information. The intellectual power of the left hemisphere lies in its ability to abstract, which can be viewed as detaching something from its context or looking at it in isolation, together with its capacity to categorize things once they have been abstracted. The right hemisphere deals with the total Gestalt, the whole being more than the sum of its parts. Specializing in nonverbal communication, it is broader in focus, such as feeling part of something larger than oneself, and is capable of frameshifts. The right understands metaphor and is concerned with social and emotional functioning and mediating new experience and information (McGilchrist, 2009).

Ultimately, one must integrate the workings of the two hemispheres. In his encyclopedic *The Master and His Emissary*, Ian McGilchrist (2009) laments that the left has seized power from the right and has blocked our needed avenues of escape – the natural world and religion – and contributed to an increasingly mechanistic and fragmented world. McGilchrist's quarrel is with excessive rationalism and Western culture's reification of the capabilities of the left hemisphere.

4 An extensive discussion on the possibility of thought transference appears in Freud (1933).

5 Balter et al. (1980) articulate that while during the psychoanalytic process both analyst and analysand are in a relaxed, less inhibited state drifting toward primary process, the analyst is less so; the analyst has the responsibility of listening and verbalizing in a therapeutic manner, which entails critical, secondary process thinking.

6 The concept transformational object (Bollas, 2011) refers to the function of the mother/early caretaker who adjusts the infant's environment to meet the infant's needs and in doing so transforms his world. Later, when the infant creates the transitional object, he is able to turn away from the caretaker and engage more with aspects of his outer environment. The fact that he is in charge of the transitional object helps lessen the loss of the original symbiotic environment. He begins to use metaphor and play with the fantasy of his own omnipotence.

However, Bollas asserts that many of us never lose our longing for the original transformational object whom we imagine can propel us toward revitalization and rebirth. There can be many shades and varieties of this longing. This wish can be positive, such as choosing a loving partner who complements the self and facilitates psychological growth. A negative example is the person obsessed with committing the perfect crime. This becomes the transformational object, as, in fantasy, the perfect crime will bring financial well-being and repair psychological deficits.

7 These anthropological issues and their relationship to neurosis are discussed in depth by Freud (1912–1913) in Totem and Taboo.

8 The literature on projective identification is vast. The term projective identification is used variously to indicate a defense, a fantasy, an attempt at communication, or an object relationship. Similarly, different motives are attributed to its use: to rid the self of unwanted aspects, to control the object, to avoid separation and to communicate a state of mind so as to be contained (Auchincloss & Samberg, 2012).

The following are some suggested readings. For an overview of the history of the concept, see Elizabeth Spillius and Edna O'Shaughnessy (2012). Although a normal and universal process in development, projective identification can indicate severe pathology when used excessively (Auchincloss & Samberg, 2012): as in borderline personality (Kernberg, 1987; McWilliams, 2011; Ripoll, 2012), extreme narcissistic retreat (Rosenfeld, 1990; Steiner, 2009; Strauss, 2012) and psychosis (Rosenfeld, 2012). It is seen in lesser disturbance as well. In fact, it can appear whenever the patient has not digested unacceptable affects and needs the therapist to facilitate bringing these to consciousness. In most instances, the patient's use of projective identification offers valuable clues to underlying issues, as long as the therapist is able to process the intense affects involved.

9 To me, the term "subjugating third" is harsh, and I prefer to view this phenomenon as a "surrendering third."

10 I am grateful to Terry Marks-Tarlow for her extensive and generous discussions regarding fractals and synchrony.

11 Basic units of the brain and nervous system, neurons are nerve cells that transmit nerve impulses throughout the body. Each neuron is composed of dendrites, an axon and a cell body. The dendrites receive messages from axons in other

neurons. The totality of messages received determine whether the neuron will be activated. If it is, an action potential is formed. This is an electrical impulse which rapidly travels down the length of the axon and releases a neurotransmitter into the synapse, facilitating communication among neurons (https://qbi.uq.edu.au/brain/brain-anatomy/what-neuron).

A synapse is the tiny space between the axon of one neuron and the dendrite of another. Neurons communicate across the synapse via various chemical neurotransmitters, such as serotonin and dopamine, which are released by the action potential. The neurotransmitters travel across the synapse and create an electrical signal to either excite or inhibit the neighboring neuron.

https://qbi.uq.edu.au/brain-basics/brain/brain-physiology/action-potentials-and-synapses

12 Mirror neurons, a type of premotor neuron, have been found in both monkeys and humans. They are activated not only when monkeys or humans execute certain actions but also *when they observe others executing similar actions* (Kilner & Lemon, 2013). Mirror neurons in the human brain have been found to play a role in understanding, without words, the intention of others (Iacoboni et al., 2005).

13 Nonlocal effects are effects at a distance, which contradicts the classical requirement of locality, that only things very close to each other can influence one another.

14 Founded in 1979 by Robert Jahn, dean emeritus of the Princeton Engineering School, and Brenda Dunne, the PEAR Laboratory was established to investigate the impact of the human mind on physical, material systems. The Laboratory closed in 2007. Dunne was formerly Laboratory manager. Jahn and Dunne are coauthors of *Margins of Reality: The Role of Consciousness in the Physical World.*

References

Ardito, R. & Rabellino, D. (2011). Therapeutic alliance and outcome of psychotherapy: Historical excursus, measurements, and prospects for research. *Frontiers in Psychology*, 2:270.

Aron, L. (1998). "Yours, thirsty for honesty": Some background to Sandor Ferenczi's pursuit of mutuality. *American Journal of Psycho-Analysis*, 58 (1):5–20.

Aron, L. (2006). Analytic impasse and the third: Clinical implications of intersubjectivity. *International Journal of Psycho-Analysis*, 87:349–368.

Auchincloss, E.L. & Samberg, E. (Eds.). (2012). *Psychoanalytic terms and concepts.* New Haven, CT: Yale University Press.

Balint, M. (1955). Notes on parapsychology and parapsychological healing. *International Journal of Psycho-Analysis*, 36:31–35.

Balter, L., Lothane, Z. & Spencer, J. (1980). On the analyzing instrument. *Psychoanalytic Quarterly*, 49:474–504.

Bass, A. (2001). It takes one to know one: Or, whose unconscious is it anyway? *Psychoanalytic Dialogues*, 11:683–702.

Beebe, B. & Lachmann, F. (2002). *Infant research and adult treatment: Co-constructing interactions.* Hillsdale, NJ: Analytic Press.

Benedetti, G. (1987). Illuminations of the human condition in the encounter with the psychotic patient. In J. Sacksteder, D.P. Schwartz & Y. Akabane (Eds.), *Attachment and the therapeutic process: Essays in honor of Otto Allen Will, Jr., M.D.* (pp. 185–196). Madison, CT: International Universities Press.

Benjamin, J. (2004). Beyond doer and done-to: An intersubjective view of thirdness. *Psychanalytic Quarterly*, 73:5–46.
Benjamin, J. (2009). A relational psychoanalysis perspective on the necessity of acknowledging failure in order to restore the facilitating and containing features of the intersubjective relationship (the shared third). *International Journal of Psycho-Analysis*, 90:441–445.
Benjamin, J. (2010). Where's the gap and what's the difference? The relational view of intersubjectivity, multiple selves, and enactment. *Contemporary Psychoanalysis*, 46:112–119.
Bion, W.R. (1959). Attacks on linking. *International Journal of Psycho-Analysis*, 40:308–315.
Blechner, M.J. (1994). Projective identification, countertransference and the "maybe-me". *Contemporary Psychoanalysis*, 30:619–630.
Bollas, C. (Ed.) (2011). The transformational object. In *The Christopher Bollas Reader* (pp. 1–12). New York: Routledge.
Bouwmeester, D., Pan, J., Mattle, K., Eidl, M., Weinfurter, H. & Zeilinger, A. (1997). Experimental quantum teleportation. *Nature*, 390:575–579.
Brabant, E., Falzeder, E. & Giampieri-Deutsch, P. (Eds.). (1993). *The correspondence of Sigmund Freud and Sandor Ferenczi*, Volume 1, 1908–1914 (F.T. Hoffer, Trans.). Cambridge, MA: Harvard University Press.
Bromberg, P. (2006). *Awakening the dreamer: Clinical journeys.* Mahwah, NJ: The Analytic Press.
Brottman, M. (2009). Psychoanalysis and magic: Then and now. *American Imago*, 66(4):471–489.
Carroll, L. (2015). *Alice's adventures in wonderland and through the looking glass.* New York: Barnes and Noble.
Drob, S.L. (2000). *Kabbalistic metaphors: Jewish mystical themes in ancient and modern thought.* Northvale, NJ: Jason Aronson.
Duray, D. (February 28, 2018). In the studio with an actress turned painter. *New York Times*, Sunday Styles Section, p. 3.
Ehrenwald, J. (1978). *The ESP experience: A psychiatric validation.* New York: Basic Books.
Epstein, S., Pacini, R., Denes-Raj, V. & Heier, H. (1996). Individual differences in intuitive-experiential and analytical-rational thinking styles. *Journal of Personality and Social Psychology*, 71:390–405.
Eshel, O. (2006). Where are you, my beloved? *International Journal of Psycho-Analysis*, 87:1603–1627.
Evans, J.S.B.T. (2003). In two minds: Dual-process accounts of reasoning. *Trends in Cognitive Science*, 7:454–459.
Falzeder, E. & Brabant, E. (Eds.). (1996). *The correspondence of Sigmund Freud and Sandor Ferenczi*, Volume 2, 1914–1919 (P.T. Hoffer, Trans.). Cambridge, MA: Harvard University Press.
Falzeder, E. & Brabant, E. (Eds.). (2000). *The correspondence of Sigmund Freud and Sandor Ferenczi*: Volume 3, 1920–1933 (P.T. Hoffer, Trans.). Cambridge, MA: Harvard University Press.
Farrell, D. (1983). Freud's 'thought-transference', repression, and the future of psychoanalysis. *International Journal of Psycho-Analysis*, 64:71–81.

Ferenczi, S. (1980). Psychogenic anomalies of voice production. In J. Richman (Ed.), *Further contributions to the theory and technique of psychoanalysis* (J. Suttie, Trans.), (pp. 105–109). London: Karnac.
Fractal Foundation online course, https://fractalfoundation.org/OFC/OFC-1-1.html
Frazer, J. (1994). R. Fraser (Ed.), *The golden bough: A study in magic and religion: A new abridgement from the second and third editions (Oxford World's Classics).* New York: Oxford University Press.
Freud, S. (1911). Psycho-analytic notes on an autobiographical account of a case of Paranoia (Dementia Paranoides). *Standard Edition*, 12:1–82.
Freud, S. (1912). Recommendations to physicians practicing psycho-analysis. *Standard Edition*, 12:111–120.
Freud, S. (1912–1913). Totem and taboo. *Standard Edition*, 13:1–161.
Freud, S. (1915). The unconscious. *Standard Edition*, 14:159–215.
Freud, S. (1919). The "Uncanny." *Standard Edition*, 17:219–252.
Freud, S. (1921). Psychoanalysis and telepathy. *Standard Edition*, 18:175–193.
Freud, S. (1922). Dreams and telepathy. *Standard Edition*, 18:195–220.
Freud, S. (1923). Two encyclopaedia articles: (A) Psycho-analysis. *Standard Edition*, 18:235–254.
Freud, S. (1925). Some additional notes upon dream interpretation as a whole. *Standard Edition*, 19:125–138.
Freud, S. (1933). Dreams and occultism. *Standard Edition*, 22:31–56.
Freud, S. (1941). Psycho-analysis and telepathy. *Standard Edition*, 18:177–193.
Gallese, V., Eagle, M.N. & Migone, P. (2007). Intentional attunement: Mirror neurons and the neural underpinnings of interpersonal relations. *Journal of the American Psychoanalytic Association*, 55(1):131–176.
Ghent, E. (1990). Masochism, submission, surrender – Masochism as a perversion of surrender. *Contemporary Psychoanalysis*, 26:108–136.
Green, A. (2004). *A guide to the Zohar.* Stanford, CA: Stanford University Press.
Hidas, G. (1993). Flowing over-transference, countertransference, telepathy: Subjective dimensions of the psychoanalytic relationship in Ferenczi's thinking. In L. Aron & A. Harris (Eds.), *The legacy of Sandor Ferenczi* (pp. 207–215). Hillside, NJ: Analytic Press.
Horvath, A.O. (2001). The alliance. *Psychotherapy: Theory, Research, Practice, Training*, 38(4):365–372.
Iacoboni, M., Molner-Szakacs, I., Gallese, V., Buccino, G., Mazziotta, J.C. & Rizzolatti, G. (2005). Grasping the intentions of others with one's own mirror neuron system. *PLoS Biology*, 3(3):e79. https://doi.org/10.1371/journal.pbio.0030079
Jahn, R.G. & Dunne, B.J. (1987). *Margins of reality: The role of consciousness in the physical world.* New York: Harcourt Brace.
Jones, E. (1957). *The life and work of Sigmund Freud: Volume 3, the Last Phase, 1919–1939.* New York: Basic Books, Inc.
Jung, C.G. (1989). A. Jaffe (Ed.), *Memories, dreams, reflections* (R. Winston & C. Winston, Trans.). New York: Random House, Vintage Books.
Kelso, S., Dumas, G. & Tognoli, G. (2013). Outline of a general theory of behavior and brain coordination. *Neural Networks*, 37:120–131.
Kernberg, O.F. (1987). Projection and projective identification: Developmental and clinical aspects. *Journal of the American Psychoanalytic Association*, 35:795–819.

Kilner, J.M. & Lemon, R.N. (2013). What we know currently about mirror neurons. *Current Biology*, 23:R1057–R1062.
Klein, M. (1946). Notes on some schizoid mechanisms. *International Journal of Psycho-Analysis*, 27:99–110.
Klein, M. (1955). *On identification. In Envy and gratitude and other works, 1946–1963.* New York: Delacorte Press/Seymour Laurence.
Knoblauch, S.H. (2005). Body rhythms and the unconscious: Toward an expanding of clinical attention. *Psychoanalytic Dialogues*, 15(6):807–827.
Kramer, R. (2003). Why did Ferenczi & Rank conclude that Freud had no more emotional intelligence than a pre-oedipal child? In C. Barbre, B. Ulanov & A. Roland (Eds.), *Creative dissent: Psychoanalysis in evolution* (pp. 23–26). New York: Praeger Publishers.
Kushner, L. & Tippet, K. (May 15, 2014). Kabbalah and everyday mysticism. Interview by K. Tippet. *On Being.*
Laing, R.D. (1969). *Self and others.* New York: Pantheon Books.
Lambert, M.J. & Barley, D.E. (2001). Research summary on the therapeutic relationship and psychotherapy outcome. *Psychotherapy: Theory, Research, Practice, Training*, 38(4):357–361.
Lazar, S. (2001). Knowing, influencing, and healing: Paranormal phenomena and implications for psychoanalysis and psychotherapy. *Psychoanalytic Inquiry*, 21:113–131.
Levine, L. (2012). Into thin air: The co-construction of shame, recognition, and creativity in an analytic process. *Psychoanalytic Dialogues*, 22(4):456–471.
Liebovitch, L. (1998). *Fractals and chaos simplified for the life sciences.* Oxford: Oxford University Press.
Limb, C.J. & Braun, A.R. (2008). Neural substrates of spontaneous musical performance: An fMRI study of jazz improvisation. *PLoS ONE*, 3(2):e1679. https://doi.org/10.1371/journal.pone.0001679
Lindley, D. (1996). *Where does the weirdness go? Why quantum mechanics is strange, but not as strange as you think.* New York: Basic Books.
Mandelbrot, B. (1977). *The fractal geometry of nature.* New York: W. H. Freeman.
Marks-Tarlow, T. (1999). The self as a dynamical system. *Nonlinear Dynamics, Psychology and Life Sciences*, 3(4):311–345.
Marks-Tarlow, T. (2002). Fractal dynamics of the psyche. In B. Goertzel & A. Combs (Eds.), *Dynamical psychology, an international, interdisciplinary e-journal of complex mental affairs.* Online. www.goertzel.org/dynapsyc/2002/FractalPsyche.htm (accessed August 10, 2007).
Marks-Tarlow, T. (2004). Semiotic seams: Fractal dynamics of reentry. *Cybernetics and Human Knowing*, 1(1):49–62.
Marks-Tarlow, T. (2008). *Psyche's veil.* New York: Routledge.
Marks-Tarlow, T. (May 6, 2018). Personal communication with author.
Marks-Tarlow, T. (2020a). A fractal epistemology for a transpersonal psychology. In T. Marks-Tarlow, Y. Shapiro, K. Wolf & H. Friedman (Eds.), *A fractal epistemology for a scientific psychology: Bridging the personal with the transpersonal* (pp. 2–32). Newcastle upon Tyne, UK: Cambridge Scholars.
Marks-Tarlow, T. (2020b). Dreams, synchrony,
and synchronicity. In T. Marks-Tarlow, Y. Shapiro, K. Wolf & H. Friedman (Eds.), *A fractal epistemology for a scientific psychology: Bridging the personal with the transpersonal* (pp. 274–302). Newcastle upon Tyne, UK: Cambridge Scholars.

Mauss, M. (2001). *A general theory of magic* (R. Brain, Trans.). London: Routledge.
Mayer, E.L. (2001). On "telepathic dreams?" *Journal of the American Psychoanalytic Association*, 49(2):629–657.
Mayer, E.L. (2007). *Extraordinary knowing: Science, skepticism, and the inexplicable powers of the human mind*. New York: Bantam Dell.
McGilchrist, I. (2009). *The master and his emissary*. New Haven, CT: Yale University Press.
McWilliams, N. (2011). *Psychoanalytic diagnosis: Understanding personality structure in the clinical process*, Second edition. New York: Guilford Press.
Milner, M. (2010). *On not being able to paint*. New York: Routledge.
Mitchell, S. (1995). Interaction in the Kleinian and Interpersonal traditions. *Contemporary Psychoanalysis*, 31:65–91.
Ogden, T.H. (1979). On projective identification. *International Journal of Psycho-Analysis*, 60:357–373.
Ogden, T.H. (1994). The analytic third: Working with intersubjective clinical facts. *International Journal of Psycho-Analysis*, 75:3–19.
Ogden, T.H. (2004). The analytic third. *Psychoanalytic Quarterly*, 73(1):167–195.
Oliveira, H.M. & Melo, L.V. (2015). Huygens synchronization of two clocks. *Scientific Reports*, 5:11548; doi: 10.1038/srep11548
Pacini, R. & Epstein, S. (1999). The relation of rational and experiential information-processing styles to personality, basic beliefs, and the ratio-bias phenomenon. *Journal of Personality and Social Psychology*, 76:972–987.
Pérez, A., Carreiras, M. & Duñabeitia, J.A. (2017). Brain-to-brain entrainment: EEG interbrain synchronization while speaking and listening. *Scientific Reports*, 7(1):4190. doi: 10.1038/s41598-017-04464-4
Radin, D. (1997). *The conscious universe: The scientific truth of psychic phenomena*. San Francisco, CA: Harper Edge.
Reik, T. (1972). *Listening with the third ear*. New York: Arena Books.
Ripoll, L.H. (2012). Empathic accuracy and borderline personality disorder. *Neuro-Psychoanalysis*, 14(2):205–217.
Rosenbaum, R. (2011). Exploring the other dark continent: Parallels between psi phenomena and the psychotherapeutic process. *Psychoanalytic Review*, 98:57–90.
Rosenfeld, H.A. (1990). A clinical approach to the psychoanalytic theory of the life and death instincts: An investigation into the aggressive aspects of narcissism. *International Journal of Psycho-Analysis*, 52:169–178.
Rosenfeld, H.A. (2012). Contributions to the psychopathology of psychotic states: The importance of projective identification in the ego structure and the object relations of the psychotic patient. In E. Spillius & E. O'Shaughnessy (Eds.), *Projective identification: The fate of a concept* (pp. 76–97). New York: Routledge.
Rosengren, K.S. & French, J.A. (2015). Magical thinking. In M. Taylor (Ed.), *The Oxford handbook of the development of imagination* (pp. 42–60). New York: Oxford University Press.
Rusbridger, R. (2012). Affects in Melanie Klein. *International Journal of Psycho-Analysis*, 93(1):139–150.
Schmeidler, G. (1966). Two horns of a dilemma in relating ESP to personality. *Corrective Psychiatry and Journal of Social Therapy*, 12:98–114.
Scholem, G. (1995). *Major trends in Jewish mysticism*. New York: Schocken Books.

Schore, A.N. (June 2006). Neurobiology and attachment theory in psychotherapy. Workshop conducted at Mount Sinai Medical Center, New York.
Searles, H.F. (1976). Transitional phenomena and therapeutic symbiosis. *International Journal of Psychoanalytic Psychotherapy*, 5:145–204.
Slavin, M. & Kriegman, D. (1998). Why the analyst needs to change. *Psychoanalytic Dialogues*, 8:247–285.
Sloman, S.A. (1996). The empirical case for two systems of reasoning. *Psychological Bulletin*, 119:3–22.
Spillius, E. & O'Shaughnessy, E. (Eds.). (2012). *Projective identification: The fate of a concept*. New York: Routledge.
Stanovich, K.E. & West, R.F. (2000). Individual differences in reasoning: Implications for the rationality debate? *Behavioral and Brain Sciences*, 23:645–726.
Stanton, M. (1990). *Sandor Ferenczi: Reconsidering active intervention*. London: Free Association Books.
Starr, K. (2008). *Repair of the soul: Metaphors of transformation in Jewish mysticism and psychoanalysis*. New York: Routledge.
Steiner, J. (2009). *Psychic retreats: Pathological organizations in psychotic, neurotic and borderline patients*. New York: Routledge.
Strauss, L. (2012). Comparing a narcissistic and an autistic retreat: 'Looking through or at the window'. *International Journal of Psycho-Analysis*, 93(1):97–116.
Subbotsky, E. (2010). *Magic and the mind: Mechanisms, functions and development of magical thinking and behavior*. New York: Oxford University Press.
Suchet, M. (2004). Whose mind is it anyway? *Studies in Gender and Sexuality*, 5(3):259–287.
Suchet, M. (2016). Surrender, transformation and transcendence. *Psychoanalytic Dialogues*, 26(6):747–760.
Sun, R., Paul Slusarz, P. & Terry, C. (2005). The interaction of the explicit and the implicit in skill learning: A dual-process approach. *Psychoanalytic Review*, 112:159–192.
Thurschwell, P. (2005). *Literature, technology and magical thinking: 1880–1920*. Cambridge: Cambridge: University Press.
West, B. (2016). *Simplifying complexity: Life is uncertain, unfair and unequal*. Sharjah: Bentham Science Publishers.
Winnicott, D.W. (1971). *Playing and reality*. London: Tavistock Publications.
Zornberg, A. & Tippet, K. (October 6, 2011). The genesis of desire. Interview by K. Tippet, *On Being*.

Chapter 4

The neuropsychology of "aha" moments[1]

Continuing with the exploration of the relational imagination and the "magic" of the psychotherapeutic encounter, this chapter explores what *does* seem like magic – that "aha" moment – the sudden insight that seems to come from nowhere. Unlike the previous chapter when the therapist seems to be reading the patient's mind, in these instances, the therapist unconsciously restructures elements already presented in the treatment and views them in a new way. As the therapy progresses, the patient will also experience these insights. However, the therapist is the catalyst and model and takes the responsibility for guiding the process.

This type of insight seems to burst forth suddenly, as the person is not aware of the unconscious activity preceding the insight. This is in contrast to problem-solving which proceeds in a conscious, step-by-step, analytical fashion. It is also in contrast to pure "gut" instinct, as the "aha" moment is preceded by considerable unconscious brain activity (Kounios & Beeman, 2009).

The "aha" insight is valuable because it fosters realizations about the self and others by bringing dissociated or repressed material into consciousness so it can be used therapeutically. This can help resolve enactments (preconscious and unconscious transference/countertransference entanglements).[2] Very importantly, when these realizations happen relatively early in an enactment, they can shorten it by serving as a form of signal anxiety, allowing the clinician and patient to reflect and gain perspective. Further, these insights bring a sense of aliveness and innovation to the therapeutic dyad, preventing a drift toward familiarity and staleness.

Many failed therapies have been discussed when the patient had not benefited from "insight" and that the entire process had been too intellectual. The term "pseudo-insight" has been used to refer to this as opposed to mutative or transformative insight (McLaughlin, 1988). James McLaughlin refers to pseudo-insight as purely intellectual understanding while mutative insight engenders new perceptions of self, conscious or unconscious, which accompany developmental advancements in psychic organization. In part a right-brain phenomenon, the "aha" moment emanates from emotional, unconscious processes, allowing psychic reorganization. Such mutative analytic work involves very real struggles around old issues, replayed in new contexts of high emotional intensity.[3]

This activity requires what I term "unconscious freedom," defined as the clinician's ability to function in the implicit or unconscious relational realm with empathy and sensitivity while remaining relatively free of anxiety. It is being able to receive the unconscious, nonverbal communication of the patient and process it out of awareness. Then, in the "aha" moment, the therapist suddenly reformulates emotional information in a new, surprising and sometimes playful way. Because the "aha" moment involves a conceptual reorganization that results in a new interpretation, it is often identified as a form of creativity (Friedman & Forster, 2005). Indeed, this is a very creative aspect of psychotherapy, in that thoughts and feelings arise from the therapist's unconscious, just like a poem or a painting arises from the artist's unconscious.

Frequently, I do not use an "aha" insight with the patient directly. Instead, I process it privately to help with countertransference difficulties so I can regain empathy, and therapy can proceed. When I do use the insight directly, I usually rework it so it is less "raw" and more usable for the patient. However, I stress to the patient that if a particular insight does not resonate, then it is either wrong or needs adjustment, and we move on to understand in a new way. My insights are offerings, with the patient deciding which to choose.

New advances in neuroscience help elucidate this emotional "aha," suggesting what is happening neuronally or "underneath" the insight as we suddenly "get" the patient. As such, we will explore what happens neuropsychologically as well as psychologically. By providing an integration of psychoanalytic thinking with neuroscience, I hope to provide a deeper understanding of emotional insight, empirical support for the imaginative skills needed and suggestions to facilitate this type of insight.

In fact, both Freud (1912), in advocating the analytic attitude of evenly hovering attention, and Bion (1967), in focusing on the present moment in a state of reverie, were prescient in terms of current neuroscience. Research has emphasized the need to focus, relax and suspend judgment to facilitate sudden insight and improvisational, creative bursts (Beeman et al., 2004; Limb & Braun, 2008; Kounios & Beeman, 2009). Creative ideas are more likely to flow when we close our eyes, stare at a wall or gaze out a window, as this shuts out external stimuli and turns our focus inward (Kounios & Beeman, 2009; Salvi et al., 2015). Insight signals in the brain are weak and need attention and focus to be recognized. When enough unconscious information has accumulated, that is, when a threshold is reached, the insight breaks through to consciousness (Kang et al., 2017).

To provide a framework, the chapter will proceed as follows: (1) identification of psychological factors that contribute to unconscious freedom with examples of "aha" moments, (2) exploration of the neuropsychological underpinnings of this type of insight and (3) suggestions for the enhancement of the emotional freedom needed to experience these insights.

Facilitating unconscious freedom and the "aha" moment

What exactly gives the therapist the freedom to be this imaginative – to be able to step out of a fixed way of thinking about a patient and arrive at a sudden emotional insight? What constitutes this type of 'therapeutic self'?

While there is now growing consensus that the therapeutic interaction is a result of the intersubjective field that is coconstructed by both participants (Mitchell, 1988; Benjamin, 1990, 2018; Ogden, 1994; Aron, 1996 and others), the therapist also needs to have a well-defined therapeutic self (Schore, 2007) so this coconstruction does not drift toward unsettling, unproductive enactments, or even more disturbingly, into chaos. The therapist strives to have the strength and balance to contain affect and retain a sense of her own subjective self while relating interactively and authentically.

This is a dual concept. The therapist must have an appropriately separate clinical self[4] yet also able to be deeply connected, as she involves herself in the synchronizations and alignments that promote relational coconstruction. She balances her emotional involvement with an ability to observe and reflect.

Together, these factors comprise the clinician's expertise which allows her to enter the patient's subjective world. From this point of view, to achieve insight, the therapist needs to be both "neat" with well differentiated boundaries and a strong sense of self but also "sloppy,"[5] that is, open and porous, in order to tolerate needed relaxation of boundaries. When either therapist or patient do become dysregulated, a sudden insight can bring clarity.

Yet in both therapist and patient, there are strong forces operating against insight. Describing a bias in the brain toward economy and efficiency, neuroscientist Gregory Berns (2008) writes the brain is programmed to view the world in familiar, unoriginal ways. This uses the least amount of energy possible, and the brain needs to be energy efficient. Therefore, as therapists, we may need a counterbias toward creativity and innovative thinking. Earl Miller and Jonathan Cohen (2001) have investigated how, on a neural basis, we use the prefrontal cortex as our orchestra leader, guiding which direction our neural activity will go, to the left hemisphere for logical thinking or to the right for holistic, insightful thinking. By inviting reverie and being receptive and open, the therapist may be able to tilt toward creative thinking.

Clinical empathy and sensitivity

Allan Schore's opus (2007, 2009, 2011, 2017, 2019 among others) provides valuable insight into the processes of clinical empathy and sensitivity,[6] both of which are required to have the flexibility and intuition necessary for emotional freedom. In the caregiver/infant relationship, the caregiver is empathically attuned to her infant through right brain-to-right brain nonverbal visual, auditory and tactile communications as the attachment bond is cocreated. During this critical period of growth of the early developing right hemisphere (Chiron et al., 1997), caregiver and infant learn the rhythmic patterns of the other and modify their behavior to fit those patterns, creating a moment-to-moment synchronized interaction, as they build the structural system of the right brain, the home of the "relational unconscious" (Schore, 2009). The sensitive caregiver regulates the infant's states of arousal. Affect regulation – critical to the organization of the self – is learned in this right brain-to-right brain dyadic situation. Oftentimes, this interaction occurs in mother-infant pairing but is also, of course, present when fathers are caregivers.

Similarly, as the therapist creates the emotional interconnection with the patient, right brain to right brain, she promotes the patient's attachment bond and ability to self-regulate. The therapist is finely attuned to slight changes in the patient's face, vocalizations and body movements. The therapist's own state changes in relationship to this, and she adjusts accordingly. On a neural level, empathy within the psychotherapeutic relationship reduces stress-induced affective arousal (Adler, 2002), creating a relaxed state of mind in both members of the dyad. These interactions facilitate an increased capacity for mutative insight in both therapist and patient.

However, at times dysregulation in the therapist due to transference/countertransference entanglements can block the therapist's empathy, eventually leading to impasse, as my example below indicates. In response to irritation and frustration, a sense of urgency developed in me, which may have led to the intense focus needed for this type of insight.

Disturbed attachment/crossover from the implicit to the explicit domain

A sudden realization came in a series of images, which brought previously dissociated or repressed material to consciousness, making the implicit explicit and resulting in greater empathy and awareness. The thoughts and images I will describe came from my unconscious processing of the problem, similar to the process described by the cognitive researchers Mark Beeman et al. (2004): a search for a solution, an impasse and then a burst of an "aha" solution. When the therapist is able to do this, the patient feels reached at a level beneath his familiar patterns.

Ms. T is a 35-year-old woman exhibiting signs of depression and anxiety.[7] She has a fraternal twin sister. Her mother had recently died of breast cancer, and one of the patient's main symptoms was an obsession with breast cancer. The patient reports that her mother had been depressed and distant for most of the patient's life. In sessions, the patient talked a great deal about her obsession: her terror and helplessness and her constant breast self-examinations and trips to doctors because she "felt something," although clinical findings were never found. The patient did not give any history of abuse.

I felt a sense of irritation and urgency developing as I listened to what seemed to be a repetitive obsessive refrain with very little ability to reflect. After listening for a number of sessions to her obsession and starting to feel somewhat abused and helpless myself by the concreteness and irrationality of the repetition, I had an image of a little girl, very stern, verbally attacking herself by being self-critical and angry. Then a horrifying image suddenly came to me. It was of a young teenager taking a sharp knife and anxiously but insistently trying to cut off her breasts. I translated this raw image into something more useable for the patient and said, "This is a self-attack on your body. Your obsession with breast cancer is self-abuse." This did surprise her enough to interrupt the obsession and make her think. It created a "gap" or space between herself and her symptom, and she began to question her obsession.

Then, fortunately, several weeks later, her sister spontaneously told her about an incident when she saw their mother beating my patient. The patient had no memory of this, but had internalized the pattern of abuse and was continuing to do this to herself with her obsessions. This new information helped her fight her masochistic tendencies, and the obsession gradually subsided.

It is likely the patient communicated her unconscious knowledge of being beaten through her self-directed hostility, conveyed by her obsession about imagined breast cancer. I unconsciously registered her communications, expressed in the anger and violence of my visual images (although I did not yet know the specifics of her being beaten). Then I translated the images into usable data for the patient. Emotional insight occurs in this moment of successful "crossover" from the implicit to the explicit.

While my anxiety and irritation originally contributed to the impasse, it also triggered its resolution. While one usually thinks of a relaxed state of mind as facilitating focus, a sense of urgency, if not too overwhelming, may also help with intense focus (Lehrer, 2008) and can facilitate an insight bursting through to consciousness.

Anxiety and dysregulation

In intense transference/countertransference entanglements when anxiety is high, therapist and patient are relating with dysregulated right hemispheres: fear system to fear system. Other times, the enactment is more subtle with less dissociation present. Either experience can interfere with the ability to think flexibly and restructure one's approach, and access to insight is blocked. The therapeutic couple temporarily loses its imagination – the ability to think and feel freely (Bass, 2003; Bromberg, 2003; Ginot, 2007, 2015).

From a neuroscientific point of view, these inflexible patterns can literally drown out emotional insight. The enactment creates too much noise for the signal (insight) to be heard, likely disrupting the right hemispheric activation necessary for insight (Beeman et al., 2004). Joseph LeDoux (1996) discusses how strong emotions (such as those from intense transference/countertransference) can easily flood consciousness and displace or prevent other ideas from awareness. However, the therapist also has the capability to pull out of the enactment and regain perspective, including when not in session. Early morning – when the brain is unwound, disorganized and open to new ideas – is an ideal time for insight (Beeman as quoted in Lehrer, 2008). The right hemisphere is also very active during this time.

Relaxation and insight

The following vignette is an insight I had about a patient on awakening. I was still in a relaxed state of mind before the stimuli of the day had a chance to intrude.

Mrs. R, in treatment for depression and anxiety, became more markedly depressed several years into treatment. She had achieved certain milestones in her life. These included success as a lawyer and her recent election to local office. Prior to this current episode of intense depression, the patient had been preoccupied with and critical of her mother's alternating rages and depression when my patient was a child. During this recent seemingly relentless depression, my patient described how she feels completely lost after work. Despite having two young children at home, she wandered aimlessly at a local suburban mall for hours after work. I found myself feeling very critical of her. Although her children were being cared for by two nannies, they needed her. I wondered why she couldn't spend that time with them, creating a better atmosphere in the home. I said something to this effect, and she understandably became quiet. Then she said she felt I was judging her. I recognized that my tone was critical. As I stepped back, I tried to get her to talk more about how depressed she feels and acknowledged her feelings of helplessness.

However, right after I woke up the morning following this therapy session, I suddenly realized we were enacting some kind of "fight." I had become provoked by her helplessness and critical of how little she could or would do. I remembered how her mother berated her when she did something contrary to her mother's demands. I then fully realized this current depression was triggering intense early memories of helplessness and anger, feelings she sought to avoid by not going home. She also very much wanted to protect her children from the escalating arguments she was beginning to have with them. She did not have any significant conflicts with them prior to her current depression.

I now viscerally understood our enactment (and hers with her children). My critical statements about her not going home immediately after work to be with her children were an example of unconscious imprisonment; I was trapped in a pattern akin to the pattern she had with her critical mother as well as aspects of my own history, and I acted it out. Close to a feeling of unconscious freedom, thoughts came quickly to me that next morning, seemingly with no preparation, and felt right. I was able to talk fruitfully with Mrs. R in subsequent sessions about how she was manifesting some of the qualities of her mother with her children and how we were also engaged in an enactment. As the patient became increasingly self-aware, she devised a method herself to stop the arguments with her children. When she would start to feel provoked, she would consciously conjure up how she felt when her mother would berate her. She could then feel greater empathy for her children, and her irritability largely subsided. She was able to reenter the very creative activity of mothering once she was more conscious of the early dysfunctional patterning of entwinement with her abusive mother.

In the above example, out of awareness my right brain was likely unconsciously processing different explanations for what happened between us and testing each explanation until it came up with the right one (Beeman et al., 2004; Lehrer, 2008). Then without consciously thinking about the patient, the correct idea came to me. Relating this realization to Mrs. R. felt easy. However, when I was trapped in the enactment, my interaction with her felt very difficult.

At first the patient dysregulated me. Then after my insight, I was able to regulate her. Although an everyday example, this is an act of unconscious freedom because I was able to release myself from the intersubjective entrapment of early emotional patterns and reframe what was happening in a new way. My clinical empathy was restored.

Allowing unformulated thoughts to surface

Continuing with the exploration of relational freedom, Donnel B. Stern (DB Stern) focuses on allowing unformulated thoughts to surface to generate new understanding. Catching glimpses of unconscious thoughts, the analyst takes the risk of playing with fleeting images to allow something unexpected, something "unbidden" (DB Stern, 1990, p. 452) to surface. One "receives" these thoughts rather than searches for them. This clinician usually evaluates and develops these unbidden thoughts before presenting them to the patient, although sometimes they are said spontaneously.

An example is as follows. After mulling it over and being uncertain, DB Stern suggested to a patient that he should have called him in a moment of distress, even though Stern doesn't usually encourage patients to call between sessions, especially when, as in this case, the anxiety has unconscious roots and is related to current themes in the treatment. However, Stern said it anyway, and the remark greatly touched the patient. Then, in the form of free associations to the patient's narrative, unbidden thoughts continued to come to Stern throughout the session, creating new intensity in the therapeutic relationship (2013b). This allowed unformulated thoughts to become formulated, including Stern and the patient emotionally realizing for the first time the depth of the patient's long-standing loneliness arising from a traumatic event when he was much younger. As Stern indicates, it can be difficult to discern whether patient or analyst first initiates the unbidden thoughts. At different moments, it can be one or the other, and unconscious factors are always at work.

The intersubjective field facilitates or prevents relational freedom (DB Stern, 2013b). One or both sides of the dyad must have an unconscious willingness to surrender to the field in order to allow the unbidden to come to consciousness. Whatever can be done, especially "courting surprise" (DB Stern, 1990, p. 452), to facilitate this process promotes therapeutic action. Conversely, rigidities and enactments in the field are destructive constraints on freedom. Clinicians need to attend to blocks in the field so therapy can proceed (DB Stern, 2013b). As relational freedom expands in both patient and analyst, novel unprompted meanings, insights and experiences appear spontaneously. For Stern, relational freedom is the bedrock of therapeutic action.

The importance of reverie

Ideally, the therapist listens with a special type of calm receptivity or reverie, a meditative-like stance. She attends to both the patient, his words and his nonverbal communications, and to herself, her inner world. This allow her to grasp implicit meanings and work with unconscious murmurings in order to communicate empathy and analytic understanding. She translates beta (nonsymbolized, persecutory elements) into alpha, increasing the patient's capacity for symbolized, meaningful experience. The therapist listens for the unexpected, something said out of context or newly introduced, that may give a clue to an underlying issue and lead the therapy in a fresh direction.

Listening in this meditative way encourages a tilt toward right hemispheric activity and the possibility of insight. Roland Grabner et al. (2007, p. 228) reports that the right hemisphere "operates in a more free-associative, primary process manner, typically observed in states such as dreaming or reverie."

In instances of therapeutic impasse, Neville Symington (1983) describes how his mind will drift and wander, and he has a sudden realization. A new feeling/thought occurs, and he is able to reposition himself in relationship to the patient and cause a positive shift. A constriction in the therapeutic process falls away, and he and the patient can proceed with exploratory work. Symington calls this "an inner act of freedom" (Symington, 1983, p. 284), occurring when something within the unconscious of the analyst suddenly shifts or changes as he pulls out of the enactment. The patient perceives this, probably unconsciously, and responds. While the analyst's verbal interpretation is essential, as it makes the shift available to consciousness, Symington emphasizes that the essential element is the inner act of the analyst. He describes this type of contact as revolutionary: a new reality develops and growth begins.

Symington gives a clue as to how this type of insight might come about. Referring to Arthur Koestler's work on the creative act of insight (1975), Symington (1987) discusses how insight is frequently the result of the intersection of two matrices, the convergence of one sphere with another, leading to a solution. Koestler describes how King Hieron of Syracuse ordered Archimedes to determine if his crown was made of gold. (The king suspected that it had been diluted with silver.) Only when Archimedes was in another setting or matrix – the public baths – did he have the insight that the water displaced by his body could be a clue. As he lowered himself into the water and saw it rise, Archimedes realized that the volume of his body was equal to the quantity of water displaced. He suddenly knew he could discover the volume of gold in Hieron's crown. He could get a gold bar the same weight as the crown and measure the amount of water it displaces. Then when he put the crown in the water, if it were pure gold, it should displace the same quantity of water as the gold bar. The two contexts intersected and facilitated the insight.

To foster "aha" moments, therapists may need to go outside of their normal arena for considering problems, as in interdisciplinary activity, explicated in Chapter 8. A further extension of this is that the therapist and patient are two distinct matrices intersecting in the therapeutic situation – challenging habitual ways of viewing the world and creating the possibility for new insights.

Continuing in the vein of gaining access to what has not yet been thought, the poetic psychoanalyst Antonino Ferro stresses the importance of reverie. Representing the calm receptive state of the mother/caretaker with her infant, reverie is a term originally adopted by Bion. In this state, the caretaker is able to take in and process her infant's distress and provide comfort and meaning. Bion adopted this term to represent the analyst's function as he processes the raw material of the patient into meaningful symbols. This is a dyadic process. The patient also processes the communications of the analyst.

Following Bion, Ferro describes how the analyst, in her reverie, is able to translate the patient's raw emotions into symbolically represented experience, termed *waking dreaming*. Since analysts (and, in time, patients) are doing this throughout the session, the entire session can be experienced as a waking dream. To help facilitate this process, the analyst can think about each comment made by the patient as beginning with "I had a dream in which …" (Ferro, 2009, p 214). This de-concretizes the language of the patient and allows for more expanded meanings, moving away from a discussion of content to focusing on developing tools for creative dreaming, feeling and thinking.

Comprising both horizontal and vertical dimensions, Ferro's concept of the field[8] is one of his most original contributions (Ferro, 2015). It encompasses the horizontal plane that contains all the splits of personality in the dyad and also the vertical history of both, including the transgenerational transmission of conflict and trauma. The most important way to listen to the contents of a session is in relation to the emotional "field." By this Ferro means that every "character" (or element the patient presents) relates to the entirety of the session or the field, also defined as "… the sum of the possible worlds of analyst and patient" (Ferro, 2009, p. 218).

These "characters" are points in the narrative that contain bundles of emotion that can be taken apart and reassembled differently so as to construct new characters.[9] For example, a patient could say she became sick from very rich food (now a character in the field) and the analyst might wonder if he had been overly interpretative and therefore overwhelming. After discussion with the patient, he adjusts accordingly, thereby creating a new, more attuned character in the field.

As the process continues and the patient's raw sensations are put into digestible form by the analyst, that is, "cooked," a word of which Ferro is fond, the patient's previously unthinkable thoughts and feelings are now in symbolic form. This containment, attunement and adjustment by the analyst gradually contributes to the patient's growth and evolution.

One of many of Ferro's startling statements is that the field itself can dream. I interpret this poetic idea to mean that analyst and patient in all of their utterances can in their reverie move the analysis forward by transforming as yet unknown emotions/thoughts into usable, interpretable form. The field dreams when the analyst is a good enough container to facilitate the patient's narrative, and when the alpha functions of the analyst, and eventually the patient's as well, bring unusable raw emotions/thoughts into being.

The analyst constantly surveys the "field" to see how it represents itself. Any element of the field, such as the patient's mention of stormy weather the night before the session, may reveal the patient's perception of the analyst. The analyst listens carefully to try to ensure neither over- nor underinterpretation, so as to keep the process of transformation alive. A passing remark from a patient a number of years ago is an example of the importance of surveying the field. As the session ended, the patient said, "What do you know about Madoff's son killing himself?" At first, I was taken aback because it seemed out of context. Then later, I realized that perhaps her own questionable financial transactions were finally beginning to be of concern to her. Possibly she was remonstrating me (and herself) for not confronting these issues sooner. Possibly she had unexpressed suicidal thoughts of her own. The "field" had so far been blocked in exploring this. I did broach this, and she slowly began to address various financial practices as well as fantasies of self-harm. In Ferro's terms, the field began to dream again or, in more mundane language, the analysis became unblocked.

Separateness and emotional insight

In the above example, I had been intertwined with the patient and may have colluded in his avoidance. Alternately, the patient was simply not ready to discuss these issues prior to this moment. Regardless, after he asked me an unexpected question, I quickly regained my "separateness" and capacity to reflect. This ability to be separate offsets an over-identification with the patient and allows the therapist to gain perspective and regulate the patient's dysregulated states and her own. The therapist knows where she ends and the patient begins – even though they are bound together in the intersubjective field.

Support for this can be found in the work of neuroscientists Vittorio Gallese (2006) and Marco Iacoboni (2008) on mirror neurons, seen by them as linked to our ability to inhabit the emotional states of others. Gallese (2006) writes that empathy is the capacity to experience what others' experience while remaining separate, that is, still attributing these experiences to others and not to the self. Similarly, when discussing the workings of mirror neurons, Iacoboni (2008) emphasized the ability of the observers to maintain their own sense of themselves as separate from the subjects they observed.

However, Symington (1986) relates the difficulty analysts sometimes have remaining appropriately separate, as there are powerful projective mechanisms operating opposing this. Under these circumstances, analysts can experience such pressure they can feel immobilized, essentially temporarily losing their imagination. It is the analyst's/therapist's constant task to understand and work with these projective identifications so as to restore her therapeutic self. Part of unconscious freedom is to be, sooner or later, relatively free of the projections of the patient. However, this is a constant cycle, likely to be repeated when projective identifications again become intense. Then once more, they must be discussed and worked through.

Insight in a dream image

The following example illustrates how my dream image helped bring dissociated affects into consciousness and allowed me to develop the separateness I needed to process the patient's communications therapeutically.

While analysts have long reported images from dreams regarding patients beginning with Freud (1900), Lawrence Brown (2007) makes the point that such dreams have tended to be seen as examples of countertransference difficulties. While that may sometimes be the case, Brown argues that these dreams may also indicate that the analyst is coming to know the patient on an unconscious level by processing the patient's implicit communications and projective identifications.

Ms. A, a 29-year-old woman, entered treatment for depression and anxiety. The following is an image from my own dream that related to Ms. A's session the day before. I awoke from a dream in which all I remembered was the chilling and dreadful image of a mermaid with the face of Joan Crawford, whom I associated with both glamour and punishment/sadism. I immediately thought of my patient who the day before had been describing her mother as a seductive, yet periodically cruel woman. Although she had been discussing this a great deal in these first few months of therapy, I had been disengaged and unable to *feel* it. Whether I was mirroring her detachment or it was my own defensiveness, or both, I do not know. However, when I woke up from the dream, I was shaken and sweating and felt horror and dread about the image. On a very visceral level, I suddenly knew what my patient felt. This gave me a sense of what could develop in the treatment, that is, how we could get into an enactment where either she or I could become the Joan Crawford-mermaid and have a punishing interaction. Instead, I was forewarned by the dream image and could move forward with more awareness of her unconscious and mine.

I can speculate about what happened. Possibly the relaxation of sleep and the reduced activity of the inhibiting prefrontal cortex allowed me to transform my amorphous feelings about the patient into a meaningful symbol. As part of this, I embodied the feelings that the patient had about her mother mingled with my own life experiences. The insight burst through in the form of the visual dream image. In a condensed way, this image described in "emotional language" the relational problems of the patient, my own issues and what could happen between us. I was then able to reflect on this image and see how it related to my patient's experience of her mother, which is also an internalized aspect of herself. This unconscious insight (the image of the mermaid) helped me understand the patient from the "inside out" (Bromberg, 1998, p. 127) and be relatively free of the possibility of enacting this. Apparently, it was only in my sleep that I was initially able to tolerate the horror of the experience of this mother.[10]

This projective identification, which I experienced in the dream image of the mermaid, was an important unconscious communication to me about the patient's internal world. When I had the visual dream image, it stood out as something separate from me, something I could reflect about rather than only unconsciously experience. This is an example of the importance of self-object differentiation in facilitating emotional understanding. It may be that my earlier detachment in the treatment was an attempt to ward off this projective identification until, finally in the dream image, I was able to bear it.

Neural correlates of the "aha"

The specificity and suddenness (the "aha") of emotional insight, as in the above example, is supported by Beeman et al. (2004) who have extensively investigated the role of the right hemisphere in solving problems using insight.[11] These researchers describe the process as follows: (1) the subject consciously focuses on the problem, (2) comes to an impasse, (3) works on it unconsciously and then (4) in a sudden burst becomes aware of the solution. This is the "aha" moment. Subjects solving problems using noninsight solutions (logical, step-by-step methods) report a gradual rather than a sudden process in coming to a solution.

However, even though the experience of insight appears to happen all at once, it is actually the end product of a number of unconscious brain processes operating at different time scales (Kounios & Beeman, 2009). My hope is that exploring these precursors can suggest approaches to facilitate psychotherapeutic insight and provide empirical support for the skills needed.

Using functional magnetic resonance imaging (FMRI), Beeman et al. (2004) found several neural correlates of insight, which were not present in subjects using a straightforward, noninsight method of solution. The researchers saw that a small fold of tissue on the surface of the right hemisphere (the right anterior superior temporal gyrus or RH aSTG) suddenly became intensely active in the second before the insight. The researchers suggest that this area "facilitates integration of information across distant lexical or semantic relations, allowing solvers to see connections that had previously eluded them" (Beeman et al., 2004, no pagination given). This activation likely corresponds to our feeling of "aha"!

Using electroencephalogram (EEG) measurement, they also observed a burst of high frequency activity (gamma rhythms) in the same area 300 milliseconds before the insight. By observing this area (the RHaSTG), the researchers actually knew *before* the subjects themselves who would have an insight! Gamma rhythm is thought to come from the binding of neurons, as cells draw themselves into a new network, in this case an "aha" moment. This is the formulation of a new idea.

There was another finding of a burst of slower, alpha-band activity measured over right occipital cortex when solving a problem with insight. When we are trying to answer a difficult question, we instinctively close our eyes or look away in order to focus and concentrate. The subjects in the experiment were told not to close their eyes or look away. This burst of alpha-band activity may be the brain's alternative way to focus; these rhythms block out extraneous stimuli by inhibiting visual inputs to the right hemisphere, reducing the possibility of distraction (Beeman et al., 2004; Kounios & Beeman, 2009). Creating a temporary reduction in interfering visual inputs, the alpha waves facilitate the retrieval of weakly-activated problem solutions in the right hemisphere. This supports Freud's direction to listen with evenly hovering attention and Bion and Ferro's emphasis on reverie. These states block out extraneous stimuli and allow deep focus and concentration.

Research findings on insight indicate that the RH carries out relatively coarse semantic coding (Chiarello et al., 1990; Beeman, 1998), which in turn produces large, weak semantic fields which overlap. The fact that the fields are weak accounts for the unconscious nature of this processing; it is not strong enough to be felt consciously until the insight bursts through to consciousness. This overlap among multiple semantic fields (Beeman et al., 1994) is helpful when bringing parts of a narrative together that are only distantly related (Beeman, 1993, Beeman et al., 2000), as therapists do in their work with patients. This again supports the importance of attuned right brain-to-right brain functioning in psychotherapy.

Another interesting finding is that subjects in a more positive mood are more likely to solve problems with insight rather than those in a neutral or negative mood (Subramaniam et al., 2009; Subramaniam & Vinogradov, 2013). Although this had previously been demonstrated on a behavioral level, Subramaniam and colleagues demonstrate how positive mood can influence cognition at the neural level. Their findings indicate that in comparison with subjects lower in positive mood, subjects higher in positive mood solved more problems in total, and many more with insight. Neurologically, the researchers found that positive mood increases activity in the anterior cingulate cortex/medial prefrontal cortex during the period immediately prior to solving a problem. The anterior cingulate cortex may facilitate the participant's ability to restructure and break the "frame." Positive mood may therefore be one factor that biases cognitive mechanisms toward insight while excessive anxiety may have the opposite effect.

These neurological results support the behavioral findings that suggest that individuals in a positive mood have more access to distant and/or unusual semantic associations and have greater cognitive flexibility[12] and creative problem-solving capacities (Subramaniam & Vinogradov, 2013).

Enhancing our capability for unconscious freedom

The development of the right hemispheric functions of the clinician, which include her clinical empathy, sensitivity and intuition, is crucial to her effectiveness. It is the right hemisphere that is dominant in the regulation of affect and bodily states. The clinician's ability to handle the patient's negative states involves the therapist's capacity to autoregulate these painful affects (Schore, 2007).

Mindfulness, that is, cultivating an attitude of attention to the present moment, to the fullness of our experience enhances the ability to self-regulate (Siegel, 2007). It is a form of internal attunement, a special form of attention that helps promote insight. As we practice mindfulness, Daniel Siegel explicates how we can enhance our own neural activity by strengthening the integrative functions of the medial prefrontal cortex (MPC). By doing so, we are stimulating the same area the jazz musicians did when they were creating (Limb & Braun, 2008), as discussed earlier. Therapists, and patients as well, may have an opportunity to optimize their access to creative insights, which rely on unconscious processes, by mindfulness practice.

Mindfulness practices include the practice of prayer, Buddhist mindfulness, meditation, yoga, tai chi chuan and qui quong. These practices help regulate our body, balance our emotions, modulate fear, increase flexibility of response and improve self-awareness and intuition. This facilitates emotional insight – possibly by a form of focus/relaxation, which allows us to block out extraneous signals, which can prevent insight.

There are varying positions on the role of the hemispheres in fear modulation, empathy, attuned communication and intuition. While Siegel stresses the integration of right and left hemispheric functions as important, Schore stresses the centrality of development of the complexity of the right hemisphere. An extensive discussion of this issue is beyond the scope of this chapter but future research is needed to refine our understanding.

There is a bidirectional aspect to this process: the mind (the psychological) can change the brain (the neurological) and the brain can change the mind. Strengthening the psychological helps us neurologically as does strengthening the neurological help us psychologically. Siegel and colleagues (Schore, 1994, 2003a,b; Siegel, 1999, 2007; Cozolino, 2002; Siegel & Hartzell, 2003; Solomon & Siegel, 2003) have proposed that an effective therapeutic relationship between clinician and patient promotes the growth of the fibers in the prefrontal area, suggesting that the therapeutic relationship can strengthen the MPC, promoting integrative and creative functioning. However, one can enhance the neural activity of the MPC directly by mindfulness practice and bring about positive psychological results. Patients and therapists can work this from either direction.

Buddhist concepts, including mindfulness, can be linked with Bion (Pelled, 2007). In both systems of thought, psychological growth is related to learning from experience. Comparing the concept of attention in Bion and the concept of mindfulness in Buddhism, Esther Pelled states that in both systems, attention must be separated from other mental processes in order to learn from experience. The reverie of Bion and the Buddhist state of equanimity are also compared. She argues that increasing the capacity for reverie is also the objective of Buddhist practice, that is, "... improving the inner container such that it can hold any content while unmoved by desire" (Pelled, 2007, p. 1507). Through focus and discipline, the mind is able to transcend its own limitations.

The "aha" insight, an aspect of the relational imagination, is an inspired, transcendent moment. We are released from restrictive thinking about the patient. This helps the dyad move toward greater analytic freedom, and new imaginative realities can be created.

Notes

1 An earlier version of this chapter appeared in Domash (2010) and is gratefully reprinted with permission from Guilford Press.
2 For a history of the concept of enactment, including controversies surrounding the term, see Ellman, S. & Moscowitz, M. (2004). *Enactment: Towards a new approach to the therapeutic Relationship.* North Bergen, NJ: Jason Aronson. See also: Aron, L. (2003). The paradoxical place of enactment in psychoanalysis. *Psychoanalytic Dialogues*, 13(5):623–631.
3 Researchers have assessed the relative accuracies of insight vs. analytic/logical solutions. They found "aha" insights are more likely to be correct, possibly because insight solutions burst into consciousness all at once when the unconscious solving process is complete. In contrast, analytic problem solvers may incorrectly offer guesses based on conscious, premature processing (Salvi et al., 2016).

When faced with a deadline (in therapy terms, possibly the end of the session) participants made different types of errors when solving a problem by insight versus logic. When using insight, the participants let the time run out (error of omission) if they didn't have an insight, while those using logic offered an incorrect answer (error of commission) rather than let the time run out (Kounios et al., 2008). This argues for the therapist to use an insight approach and wait for the right moment rather than feel she *has* to offer a logical response, which may be premature and out of step with the patient.
4 By "clinical self," I am indicating the totality of the therapeutic abilities of the therapist, how she uses her "self" clinically.
5 Applying dynamical systems theory to psychoanalysis, the Boston Change Process Study Group (BCPSG) coined the term "sloppiness" to refer to the unpredictable and improvisational aspects of the therapeutic process, including how each member has to infer the meaning in the communication of the other. This creates variability, unpredictability, uncertainty and surprise, and the possibility of generating new thought (DN Stern et al., 1998; Nahum, 2005). I am using the term "sloppy" somewhat differently here to highlight the importance of the therapist having open and porous boundaries in the interest of creative coconstruction while paradoxically being neat and differentiated at the same time.
6 Schore (2007) defines sensitivity as the clinician's ability to receive and express nonverbal affective communications and defines empathy as the clinician's right brain activity within the subjective field. We gather our data for emotional insight from our clinical sensitivity and clinical empathy.
7 This example appeared in Leanne Domash (2009).
8 Ferro and DB Stern's conception of the field have similarities and differences. Both favor experience-near understanding and place an emphasis on affect. For both, symbolic experience may not have been formed but rather exists as a potential not yet actualized. In classical analysis, the unconscious is repressed but waiting to be recovered once defenses are analyzed.

Although both Ferro and DB Stern favor experience that is cocreated, what is cocreated is different (DB Stern, 2013a). An interaction of unconscious fantasies with little reference to external reality, Ferro's concept of the field is not a combination of inner and outer reality but inner and inner – the internal, fantasy worlds of analyst and patient. The analyst contains the patient and through her reverie, transforms the patient's primitive mentalizations into symbolically represented experience. The relational position, on the other hand, is dialectical. The inner and outer world (and their continuous interaction) of both analyst and patient constitute one of the most significant dialectical pairs in creating the intersubjective field (DB Stern, 2013a).

9 Ferro uses language from narrative theory, which studies how people develop stories to understand their world. Narration is a strategy for coming to terms with experience in contrast to other methods, such as poetry, argument, scientific discourse, etc. Narratives are ubiquitous, appearing in literary fiction and nonfiction, courtrooms, doctors' offices and, of course, in psychotherapy (see https://projectnarrative.osu.edu/about/what-is-narrative-theory).

Ferro emphasizes the narration of the patient and the "characters," which can be any element in the story, that arise in the narration. When new "characters" appear, that is an indication of an expansion of the subjectivity of the patient. Like directors who move the story forward, analysts work with characters already present and help the patient introduce new characters to promote narrative development and transformation (Choder-Goldman, 2016).

10 Research indicates that during dreaming the amygdala, the fear activation center, is very active in creating our unconscious emotional reality and the frontal cortex relatively inactive. During dreaming we can get a glimpse of our terror without the regulating, inhibitory effect of the prefrontal cortex (Goleman, 2003).

11 A possible limitation to using Beeman and colleagues' work to understand psychotherapy is that their subjects were solving verbal problems adapted from a test of creative cognition, not problems arising from working psychotherapeutically. Beeman et al. (2004) used a set of compound remote association problems. Subjects saw 3 problem words, namely, pine, crab and sauce, and had to supply the one word that can form a familiar compound word with each of the 3 problem words, such as apple to make pineapple, crabapple and applesauce. However, even though the task of Beeman's subjects and the task of the therapist are different, I suggest we can learn something from their work about the process of insight in the therapeutic situation. What brings the analytic insight to consciousness may be the same process as for Beeman's subjects. LeDoux (1996) writes that the same mechanism of consciousness brings both cognitive and emotional stimuli to consciousness, although the systems that provide the inputs to the mechanism of awareness differ.

This is even more probable since as Beeman (2004, 2005) reports, this same area in the right hemisphere increases in activity when people comprehend complex, natural language (Beeman, 2005), during tasks that emphasize integration across sentences to extract themes (St. George et al., 1999) and when subjects are asked to form more coherent memories for stories (Mason & Just, 2004). This is similar to the activity of clinicians, listening to patients' complex stories and extracting themes. Beeman's work suggests that to the extent therapists can allow their right hemisphere to solve problems, trusting it to function out of awareness, and not rely on their left brain's need to "solve" the problem logically, then they are more likely to have emotional insight. In fact, Schooler et al. (1993) have shown how it is possible to override insight solutions by asking participants to explain or put into words how they solve problems.

12 In trying to solve a problem with insight, the person frequently comes to an impasse. Flexibility, including the ability to switch strategies and find alternative solutions, is needed to overcome the impasse. The problem solver must be able to move away from what is habitual but not working and gain access to more distant but applicable concepts. Then frequently, she can recognize connections

and find the solution. The is the "aha" moment (Subramaniam et al., 2009; Subramaniam & Vinogradov, 2013).

References

Adler, H.M. (2002). The sociophysiology of caring in the doctor–patient relationship. *Journal of General Internal Medicine*, 17:883–890.

Aron, L. (1996). *A meeting of minds: Mutuality in psychoanalysis.* Hillsdale, NJ: The Analytic Press.

Bass, A. (2003). "E" Enactments in psychoanalysis: Another medium, another message. *Psychoanalytic Dialogues*, 13(5):657–675.

Beeman, M.J. (1993). Semantic processing in the right hemisphere may contribute to drawing inferences from discourse. *Brain Language*, 44:80–120.

Beeman, M.J. (1998). Coarse semantic coding and discourse comprehension. In M.J. Beeman & C. Chiarello (Eds.), *Right hemisphere language comprehension: Perspectives from cognitive neuroscience* (pp. 255–284). Mahwah, NJ: Lawrence Erlbaum Associates.

Beeman, M.J. (2005). Bilateral brain processes for comprehending natural language. *Trends in Cognitive Sciences*, 9(11):512–518.

Beeman, M.J., Bowden, E.M. & Gernsbacher, M.A. (2000). Right and left hemisphere cooperation for drawing predictive and coherence inferences during normal story comprehension. *Brain Language*, 71:310–336.

Beeman, M., Bowden, E., Haberman, J., Frymiare, J., Arambel-Liu, S., Greenblatt, R., Reber, P. & Kounios, J. (2004). Neural activity when people solve verbal problems with insight. *PLoS Biol*, 2(4):e97. doi: 10.1371/journal.pbio.0020097

Beeman, M.J., Friedman, R.B., Grafman, J., Perez, E., Diamond, S. & Lindsay, M.B. (1994). Summation priming and coarse semantic coding in the right hemisphere. *Journal of Cognitive Neuroscience*, 6:26–45.

Benjamin, J. (1990). An outline of intersubjectivity: The development of recognition. *Psychoanalytic Psychology*, 7(Suppl):33–46.

Benjamin, J. (2018). *Beyond doer and done to: Recognition theory, intersubjectivity and the third.* New York: Routledge.

Berns, G. (2008). *Iconoclast: A neuroscientist reveals how to think differently.* Boston, MA: Harvard Business Press.

Bion, W. (1967). Notes on memory and desire. *Psychoanalytic Forum*, 2:271–280.

Bromberg, P.M. (1998). *Standing in the spaces: Essays on clinical process, trauma, and dissociation.* Hillsdale, NJ: Analytic Press.

Bromberg, P.M. (2003). One need not be a house to be haunted. *Psychoanalytic Dialogues*, 13(5):689–709.

Brown, L.J. (2007). On dreaming one's patient: Reflections on an aspect of countertransference dreams. *Psychoanalytic Quarterly*, 76(3):835–886.

Chiarello, C., Burgess, C., Richards, L. & Pollock, A. (1990). Semantic and associative priming in the cerebral hemispheres: Some words do, some don't … sometimes, some places. *Brain Language*, 38:75–104.

Chiron, C., Jambaque, I., Nabbout, R., Lounes, R., Syrota, A. & Dulac, O. (1997). The right brain hemisphere is dominant in human infants. *Brain*, 120:1057–1065.

Choder-Goldman, J. (2016). A conversation with Antonino Ferro. *Psychoanalytic Perspectives*, 13(1):129–143.

Cozolino, L. (2002). *The neuroscience of psychotherapy: Building and rebuilding the human brain*. New York: Norton.
Domash, L. (2009). The emergence of hope: Implicit spirituality in treatment and the occurrence of "psychoanalytic luck." *Psychoanalytic Review*, 96:35–54.
Domash, L. (2010). Unconscious freedom and the insight of the analyst: Exploring neuropsychological processes underlying "aha" moments. *Journal of the American Academy of Psychoanalysis and Dynamic Psychiatry*, 38:315–340.
Ferro, A. (2009). Transformations in dreaming and characters in the psychoanalytic field. *International Journal of Psycho-Analysis*, 90:209–230.
Ferro, A. (2015). *Torments of the soul: Psychoanalytic transformations in dreaming and narration* (I. Harvey, Trans.). New York: Routledge.
Freud, S. (1900). The interpretation of dreams. *Standard Edition*, 4/5:1–627.
Freud, S. (1912). Recommendations to physicians practicing psycho-analysis. *Standard Edition*, 12:111–120.
Friedman, R.S. & Forster, J. (2005). Effects of motivational cues on perceptual asymmetry: Implications for creativity and analytical problem solving. *Journal of Personality and Social Psychology*, 88:263–275.
Gallese, V. (2006). Intentional attunement: Embodied simulation and its role in social cognition. In M. Mancia (Ed.), *Psychoanalysis and neuroscience* (pp. 269–301). Milan: Springer.
Ginot, E. (2007). Intersubjectivity and neuroscience: Understanding enactments and their therapeutic significance within emerging paradigms. *Psychoanalytic Psychology*, 24:317–332.
Ginot, E. (2015). *The neuropsychology of the unconscious: Integrating brain and mind psychotherapy*. New York: Norton.
Goleman, D. (2003). *Destructive emotions? How can we overcome them?* New York: Bantam Books.
Grabner, R.H., Fink, A. & Neubauer, A.C. (2007). Brain correlates of self-related originality of ideas: Evidence from event-related power and phase-locking changes in the EEG. *Behavioral Neuroscience*, 121:224–230.
Iacoboni, M. (2008). *Mirroring people: The new science of how we connect with others*. New York: Farrar, Straus & Giroux.
Kang, Y.H.R., Petzschner, F.H., Wolpert, D.M. & Shadlen, M.N. (2017). Piercing of consciousness as a threshold-crossing operation. *Current Biology*, 27(15):2285–2295.
Koestler, A. (1975). *The act of creation*. London: Picador, Pan Books.
Kounios, J. & Beeman, M. (2009). The Aha! moment: The cognitive neuroscience of insight. *Current Directions in Psychological Science*, 18(4):210–216.
Kounios, J., Fleck, J.I., Green, D.L., Payne, L., Stevenson, J.L., Bowden, E.M. & Jung-Beeman, M. (2008). The origins of insight in resting-state brain activity. *Neuropsychologia*, 46:281–291.
LeDoux, J.E. (1996). *The emotional brain: The mysterious underpinnings of emotional life*. New York: Touchstone.
Lehrer, J. (July 28, 2008). The Eureka Hunt. *The New Yorker*, pp. 40–45.
Limb, C.J. & Braun, A.R. (2008). Neural substrates of spontaneous musical performance: An fMRI study of jazz improvisation. *PLoS ONE*, 3(2):e1679. https://doi.org/10.1371/journal.pone.0001679

Mason, R. & Just, M. (2004). How the brain processes causal inferences in text: A theoretical account of generation and integration component processes utilizing both cerebral hemispheres. *Psychological Science*, 14:1–7.

McLaughlin, J.T. (1988). The analyst's insights. *Psychoanalytic Quarterly*, 57:370–389.

Miller, E.K. & Cohen, J.D. (2001). An integrative theory of prefrontal cortex function. *Annual Review of Neuroscience*, 24:167–202.

Mitchell, S. (1988). *Relational concepts in psychoanalysis*. Cambridge, MA: Harvard University Press.

Nahum, J. (2005). The "something more" than interpretation revisited: Sloppiness and co-creativity in the psychoanalytic encounter. *Journal of the American Psychoanalytic Association*, 53:693–729.

Ogden, T.H. (1994). The analytic third: Working with intersubjective clinical facts. *International Journal of Psycho-Analysis*, 75:3–10.

Pelled, E. (2007). Learning from experience: Bion's concept of reverie and Buddhist meditation: A comparative study. *International Journal of Psycho-Analysis*, 88:1507–1526.

Salvi, C., Bricolo, E., Franconeri, S.L., Kounios, J. & Beeman, M. (2015). Sudden insight is associated with shutting out visual inputs. *Psychonomic Bulletin & Review*, 22(6):1814–1819.

Salvi, C., Bricolo, E., Kounios, J., Bowden, E. & Beeman, M. (2016). Insight solutions are correct more often than analytic solutions. *Thinking & Reasoning*, 22(4):443–460.

Schooler, J.W., Ohlsson, S. & Brooks, K. (1993). Thoughts beyond words: When language overshadows insight. *Journal of Experimental Psychology: General*, 122(2):166–183.

Schore, A.N. (1994). *Affect regulation and the origins of the self: The neurology of emotional development*. Hillsdale, NJ: Erlbaum.

Schore, A.N. (2003a). *Affect regulation and the repair of the self*. New York: W.W. Norton.

Schore, A.N. (2003b) *Affect dysregulation and disorders of the self*. New York: W.W. Norton.

Schore, A.N. (2007). Special section: Psychoanalytic research: Progress and process. Notes from Allan Schore's groups in developmental affective neuroscience and clinical practice. *Psychologist Psychoanalyst*, 27(3):6–15.

Schore, A.N. (August 8, 2009). The paradigm shift: the right brain and the relational unconscious. In Invited plenary address, 2009 Convention of the American Psychological Association, Toronto, Canada.

Schore, A.N. (2011). The right brain implicit self lies at the core of psychoanalytic psychotherapy. *Psychoanalytic Dialogues*, 2:75–100.

Schore, A.N. (2017). Playing on the right side of the brain: An interview with Allan N. Schore. *American Journal of Play*, 9(2):105–142.

Schore, A.N. (2019). *Right brain psychotherapy*. New York: Norton.

Siegel, D.J. (1999). *The developing mind: How relationships and the brain interact to shape who we are*. New York: Guilford Press.

Siegel, D.J. (2007). *The mindful brain*. New York: Norton.

Siegel, D.J. & Hartzell, M. (2003). *Parenting from the inside out: How a deeper understanding can help you raise children who thrive*. New York: Penguin Putnam.

Solomon, M.F. & Siegel, D.J. (Eds.). (2003). *Healing trauma: Attachment, mind, body, brain*. New York: Norton.

St. George, M., Kutas, M., Martinez, A. & Sereno, M.I. (1999). Semantic integration in reading: Engagement of the right hemisphere during discourse processing. *Brain*, 122:1317–1325.

Stern, D.B. (1990). Courting surprise – Unbidden perceptions in clinical practicel. *Contemporary Psychoanalysis*, 26:452–478.

Stern, D.B. (2013a). Field theory in psychoanalysis, part 2: Bionian field theory and contemporary interpersonal/relational psychoanalysis. *Psychoanalytic Dialogues*, 23(6):630–645.

Stern, D.B. (2013b). Relational freedom and therapeutic action. *Journal of the American Psychoanalytic Association*, 61(2):227–255.

Stern, D.N., Sander, L., Nathan, J., Harrison, A., Bruschweiler-Stern, N. & Tronick, E. (1998). Non-interpretative mechanisms in psychoanalytic therapy: The 'something more' than interpretation. *International Journal of Psycho-Analysis*, 79:903–921.

Subramaniam, K., Kounios, J., Parrish, T.B. & Jung-Beeman, M. (2009). A brain mechanism for facilitation of insight by positive affect. *Journal of Cognitive Neuroscience*, 21:415–432.

Subramaniam, K. & Vinogradov, S. (August 7, 2013). Improving the neural mechanisms of cognition through the pursuit of happiness. *Frontiers in Human Neuroscience*, 7:1–11.

Symington, N. (1983). The analyst's act of freedom as agent of therapeutic change. *International Review Psycho-Analysis,* 10:283–291.

Symington, N. (1986). *The analytic experience.* New York: St. Martin's Press.

Symington, N. (1987). The sources of creativity. *American Imago*, 44(4):275–287.

Chapter 5

The biology of imagination

We can learn about the improvisational, emergent and transformative aspects of the creative process by traveling to the microworld of the cell and the macroworld of evolution. This chapter explores imaginative activities at the cellular level in the body and creative processes in the grand sweep of evolution.

Biologically, we are primed to be imaginative. Simple cells in our bodies perform adaptive maneuvers that mirror the activity of our conscious minds as we solve problems and adjust to changing circumstances. The body has tremendous flexibility. We get cut. We heal. We get a cold. We get better. We get an infection. We fight it. Our DNA[1] becomes damaged. We repair it (in many cases). We have a deficit. We compensate. Even our immune system can learn. And these are not rote responses. Our body frequently responds in original ways to solve problems. Much of this happens spontaneously and automatically.[2] In part, this chapter explicates how imaginative, inventive and resourceful we are at our core.

Even though evolution lacks the foresight and intentionality of human creativity, we see aspects of a creative process at work. A very slow, step-by-step transformative process through the course of billions of years, evolution has produced an enormous variety of successful living forms, including, of course, human beings. Richard Dawkins (1996) describes how each generation of living organisms is built on the prior generation, a process called cumulative selection, an evolving, emergent process where the fittest are chosen in terms of survival and reproduction. Emergent, in this context, does not mean a sudden change but rather that new forms emerge or arise from cumulative selection.

Through the process of meiosis (formation of the sperm and egg in humans), genes[3] (fundamental units of heredity) and chromosomes[4] (long threadlike structures containing thousands of genes) provide the tremendous variety necessary for evolution to do its work. Further, in the split second that a sperm penetrates an egg, we see evolutionary design on a microlevel. During the process of fertilization, many sperm die in the acidic vaginal canal or swim in the wrong direction, including toward the other fallopian tube. Among the sperm that reach the egg, some die as they dissolve the outer membrane of the egg, preparing the way for the next sperm in line to penetrate. The sperm that penetrates the egg is certainly the fittest in the sense it is one that has survived all of these processes. There is also new evidence to suggest that, in some cases, the egg actually woos the *fittest* sperm, although the mechanism by which this happens is not clear (Nadeau, 2017).

My goal is to play with ideas in the neighboring fields of biology and evolution to see analogies and integrative opportunities for our work. I invite the imaginative therapist and her patient into this richness and creativity. While it is important to remember that borrowing a paradigm from another field can lead to awkward "mixed metaphors," there is an equal danger in *not* going outside the field to find analogies, gain perspective, deepen understanding and spark imagination. Otherwise, psychotherapy can become myopic and dogmatic. A judicious balance of stability (remaining inside the field) and variation (going to adjacent fields) is needed.

Biological building blocks of the imagination: the microworld of the neuron

Outlining the neurological basis of imagination, neurophilosopher John Kaag (2008, 2014) locates imagination in the physicality we all possess and asserts that it is wired into our nervous system. This is a process common to us all as we negotiate and adapt to changing environments. As Kaag notes, Donald Hebb's rule (1949) – neurons that fire together wire together – is relevant in that it establishes change and development as central features of the nervous system, an echo of the spontaneity and creativity associated with the imagination. Kaag maintains that the same plasticity and spontaneity characteristic of fine art and refined thought is present at the neuronal level. This same plasticity and spontaneity is also evident in good psychotherapy.

Neuroplasticity

Two examples of neuroplasticity are reentry and degeneracy. These are neural processes that allow a creative adjustment to new circumstances, the workings of the biological imagination. In suggesting that imagination is intricately connected to the body, Kaag takes a step in revising the Cartesian legacy of separation of mind and body.

Reentry, an imaginative coordination process by which the brain synchronizes separate neural maps to create new sensory and conceptual meanings, takes past forms and combines them in unique ways as well as refines preexisting patterns. Kaag refers to biologist Gerald Edelman (1987, 1999) who defines reentry as a recurring process that mediates between past patterns but also responds to the novel and problematic environmental conditions that arise. Neural maps continue to adapt, taking advantage of their latent organizational possibilities. Kaag (2008, p. 183) writes, "Edelman suggests that reentry is the neurophysiological foundation of the 'remembered present' that defines human consciousness," that is, we are aware of the past as we adjust to the present. Reentry does not progress in a predetermined manner. It cannot be predicted or fully described, exhibiting a type of plasticity that can be seen as uniquely imaginative.

To explain the concept of reentry, Kaag invokes the improvisation of jazz musicians. Each player listens to his own music but also works to combine his music with that of the other players. Kaag explains, "Each new signal causes a wave of novel sounds that, in the midst of novelty, maintains harmony with past forms" (2008, p. 183). Gradually, specific themes develop as the musicians are able to integrate each other's sounds and make a new piece of music that none of them could have created separately. Novelty and continuity are its defining mark. Stability and change – durability and flexibility – are necessary for optimal adaptation. Similarly, therapists can cultivate improvisation with their patients (Ringstrom, 2001) to create new, authentic patterns while retaining the patient's continuity with his past.

Biological examples of reentry abound as latent potentials are utilized to create new brain architecture. If a middle finger is removed, patterns in the cortex that map sensory inputs from fingers change. The neural spaces for the ring and index finger become larger and help substitute for the loss of the middle finger (Fox, 1984). A more recent review article by Daniel Feldman and Michael Brecht (2005) outlines various research on the neuroplasticity of the somatosensory cortex[5] detailing how sensory maps in the neocortex adaptively alter to reflect recent experience and learning. Kaag comments that this neuroplastic process coincides with a type of behavioral novelty, the ability to conduct new activities in light of unprecedented environmental circumstances. This again suggests that the ability to have novel responses is grounded in the neural circuitry of our nervous systems. Therapists utilize this capacity to help patients develop novel responses to long-standing problems.

I think of my patient Maria, a 40-year-old woman who as a child suffered prolonged separation from her parents due to political persecution. The following vignettes illustrate a form of "psychological" reentry, improvisational moments of connection between patient and therapist. It was summer, and the air conditioning was broken in the previous session. When she came to the next session and saw the window open a few inches, she said, "What? Still broken?" I said no, it had been fixed but I do both, turn on the air conditioning and also leave the window a little open. (I or, I should say, **we** both need as much breath or spirit as possible). She said, oh, she is very stingy and is always telling her family, especially her son, to close all the windows if the A/C is on.

Later in the session, she discussed how she has never been able to get angry with her mother for "giving her up" for a period of time to protect her. Maria felt quite numb in relation to memories of her mother. In fact, very little appeared to move her or be of importance to her. I thought of the word "stingy" she used at the start of the session and asked her if maybe she is being stingy with her anger, as to do otherwise would be to acknowledge the depth of the importance of her mother, and how vulnerable and bereft she felt without her. (I "riffed" on, or associated to, the word stingy.) The patient also enacted this stinginess with me by frequently reiterating how little the treatment means to her, how if she left she would not miss it, how much it costs, how she looks forward to my vacations and so on. Acknowledging anger at her mother, or toward me, would indicate our importance to her, and give us dangerous power over her. She would care and could be disappointed. She seemed to consider this, or at least not discount it. Toward the end of the session, she indicated that she is starting to feel a change within her. She said she can now speak more "loosely" to me, that is, not in a strictly dry and logical manner. At first, I misunderstood and said, "You mean like we have our own private language?" She was emphatic. No, it is her language but now she knows I will understand. She said she used to be grandiose and think no one could "follow" her. Now she knew I was able to and found it much more relaxing. She frequently referred to her numbness as a "wall." She said a few blocks have come down, and she felt a sense of excitement and greater expanse. The patient was beginning to tentatively feel a deeper sense of connection in the treatment.

A second important neuroplastic process is that of degeneracy, which in differential calculus refers to equations that have a common solution. Gerald Edelman and Giulio Tononi (2000) apply this concept to biology, referring to the ability of components with differing structures to achieve similar outcomes. This means that neuronally there are many pathways that can accomplish the same end, giving the system durability yet flexibility and adaptability. Kaag (2008) cites several examples. In the immune system, different antibodies can attack the same foreign invader. Similarly, different groups of genes can create the same physical characteristic of an organism, such as eye color.

Kaag gives the everyday example of a degenerate key system in which structurally dissimilar keys can open the same door. In an apartment building, each tenant's own key can be fashioned to open the common storage room, even though each key is different. Therefore, structures which are different (each tenant has a different key) can carry out the same function (open the common storage room). These two processes, reentry and degeneracy, contribute to clarifying how the mind can be both stable and flexible in an environment that is always changing.

Similarly, in work with patients, flexibility and stability intertwine. Many different approaches may work to solve a problem. Patients and therapists continue to learn which "key" unlocks the issue. Frequently, as in the degenerate key system above, several will. Patients also retain continuity, that is, a stable core of personality, as therapists help them respond in novel ways to emotional and environmental challenges.

Continuing with the discussion of neuroplasticity, Norman Doidge (2007, 2015) outlines how the brain can change its structure through thought and activity, and how the damaged brain can often reorganize itself so that when one part fails, another can adapt and substitute. As a dramatic example, Doidge (2007) describes Michelle, who was born with only half a brain. Her left hemisphere never developed, yet the brain is so capable of alteration and change that her right hemisphere adaptively took over many of the functions of the left, such as speech and language. Although she definitely has some disabilities, she functions fairly well. She is able to read, speak normally except when frustrated and hold down a part-time job. Although prone to tantrums, she is able to work hard at controlling them. She has difficulty with abstract thinking, but she is also a savant with some extraordinary mental abilities, such as memory for dates and understanding the patterning of calendars. Going back at least 18 years, she can very quickly tell you the day of the week for a particular date. Taking more time, she can go back even farther. Finally, she is able to use her imagination to heal some of her emotional pain. She imagines an afterlife, where she will be "upstairs" in heaven where she can live with other women but her parents will live nearby, where she can eat all the food she wants because it is both fat and calorie free, and where she wouldn't need money to pay for things. She is able to imaginatively self-soothe.

Mirror neurons

Another example of the biological imagination is the work of Gallese and others on the mirror neuron system, discussed previously (Gallese, 1996; Umiltà et al., 2001; Rizzolatti & Craighero, 2004; Gallese et al., 2007). These are a set of neurons in the premotor cortex of humans and monkeys[6,7] that provide a near instantaneous response on an unconscious level to both external and internal cues. Kaag (2008, p. 192) terms the workings of the mirror neuron system "imaginative adaptation," and this system contributes to our ability to have empathy, which aids our ability to adjust and relate.

To review, when one watches someone performing an action, the same neurons fire in his brain as in the brain of the person performing the action. One can then grasp the intention of the other and adapt. In addition, when animals observed only a small snippet of an action, the output in the mirror neuron system was the same as when they saw the whole action (Umiltà et al., 2001). This indicates a physiological process that allows generalizations to be made from partial observations. Kaag suggests that the work by Umiltà et al. provides an understanding of the neuronal structure that allows for hypothesis formation, a key to expanding the imagination.

Unfortunately, many patients have learned negative patterning, that is, they have witnessed or experienced destructive actions and internalized and generalized these patterns. However, mimesis – the ability to imitate or represent – also gives them the opportunity to learn new patterning. A specialized technique of dreamwork, Embodied Imagination, discussed in the next chapter, explores this possibility. Through the process of mimesis, the dreamer embodies, that is, senses in her body, various select images in her dream. These images are then formed into a composite which the dreamer mentally practices after the session. As she does so, she is likely activating mirror neurons and priming herself to learn new patterns from the images and their unique combination.

It should be emphasized that knowledge of the mirror system in humans is still in the early stages. In part because mirror neurons are so intriguing, the power and scope of this system may have been exaggerated. These cells have even been credited with influencing civilization and the development of human culture. However, the activity of mirror neurons can be altered by simple and brief training tasks. Rather than influencing culture, these cells are just as likely to have been influenced by it (Jarrett, 2013). These exaggerations may also reflect the human need to anthropomorphize and/or find meaning in biological processes.

In a review article James Kilner and Roger Lemon (2013) give evidence on what is known to date. An interesting finding in monkeys is that the actions of mirror neurons can be affected by such factors as the reward value of the observed action or the overall goal of an action. Therefore, in addition to sensory stimuli, formulations originating in other parts of the brain concerning the *meaning* of the observed behavior can also activate mirror neurons, suggesting mirror neurons are part of a complicated pattern of brain activity, not themselves the start of a causal path (Jarrett, 2013). Research does appear to indicate that mirror neurons support our empathic abilities but they are part of a complex system and do not act alone. Another issue is that the term mirror neuron refers to an array of cell types with differing activation patterns.

Psychotherapy changes the brain

In part, neuroplasticity is what allows psychotherapy to work. Eric Kandel, recipient of the 2000 Nobel Prize in Physiology and Medicine, writes that psychotherapy presumably creates long-term change through learning. Psychotherapy alters the brain "... by producing changes in gene expression that alter the strength of synaptic connections and structural changes that alter the anatomical pattern of interconnections between nerve cells of the brain" (Kandel, 1998, p. 460). Susan Vaughn, a psychoanalyst and student of Kandel's, describes a psychoanalyst as a "microsurgeon of the mind" who helps patients make needed alterations in neuronal networks (Vaughn, 1997, p. 3). As Vaughn (1997, p. 68) explains:

> Kandel and his colleagues believe that genetic and developmental factors determine the pre-existing connections among neurons in many parts of the brain but leave unspecified the strength with which (and even whether or not) many other connections will be made. When we learn, we change the long-term efficacy of synaptic connections. We alter the effectiveness of already existing pathways by changing the patterns of strength between neurons. And we form new pathways by arborizing our existing neural trees, sprouting new branches, which give rise to new neural connections.

It is interesting that Freud (1895) identified the synapse, the minute space between two neurons across which impulses pass, several years prior to Sir Charles Sherrington, who is given credit for its discovery. Foreshadowing Kandel's research, Freud even indicated that synapses might be changed by learning. Freud also began suggesting ideas about neuroplasticity. In 1888, he discussed the concept that neurons that fire together wire together, many years before Hebb (Doidge, 2007). Freud termed this the law of association by simultaneity, meaning that when two ideas are put together in consciousness, they get associated in the neuronal connections in the brain. This led to Freud's idea of free association based on the notion that our mental associations are expressions of connections created in our memory networks. He found that if he refrained from intervening, many connections, including disavowed feelings, will spontaneously come into the patient's mind. Neurons that fired together years before became wired together, and these connections appear in the patient's free associations (Doidge, 2007).

Another of Freud's important ideas is the plasticity of memory. Memory traces can be rearranged in accordance with new circumstances: a retranscription. Freud wrote in 1896, "... memory is not present once but many times over" (Mason, 1985, p. 207). However, in order for memories to be retranscribed, the patient would have to make them the focus of his conscious attention. Freud proposed the idea of transference. He explained that if he pointed out to the patient what was happening in the transference and the patient was paying close attention, the associated memories could be changed or retranscribed.

There are two memory systems and both get changed in therapy. Procedural or implicit memory, automatic and generally unconscious, is dominant in the first three years of life. Conscious explicit memory, associated with language, begins to come online in year three. If a person had a disturbance or trauma very early, then therapy can help him put his unconscious procedural memories into words and context. This fosters retranscription, especially in light of a more mature ego. The patient is then less likely to automatically "relive" or reenact the traumatic early memories. When this process is successful, the patient is able to unwire the original connections made during the trauma and alter his current pattern (Doidge, 2007), that is, interrupt rigid reenactments. In this way, psychotherapy restores the imagination.

To illustrate, Doidge gives the example of Mr. L whose mother died when he was 26 months old (Doidge, 2007). Although Mr. L denied that her death affected him, he suffered from depression and haunting dreams of searching for something he was not even sure he had lost. Very dissociated, he did not consciously connect this to his mother. Slowly, through the analysis of dreams, interpretation of transference and help with self-regulation, he began to understand he was no longer that same helpless child and became less overwhelmed. He was able to connect his desperate searching with its true trigger, the loss of his mother, and to realize that he still linked separation with death, explaining his severe depressions when treatment was interrupted. Mr. L went through a long treatment to achieve lasting change, including unlearning old patterns (unwiring old connections) and learning new ones (wiring new connections).

Teaching the immune system

Just as the brain/mind is plastic and can learn in psychotherapy, the immune system can learn and evolve. Immunotherapy is a treatment developed to help the body's own natural defense system fight diseases, such as cancer. Jim Allison MD, corecipient of the 2018 Nobel Prize in Medicine and Physiology, has been a pioneer in immune checkpoint therapy (Sharma & Allison, 2015). It developed from Allison's basic science research with T cells, a type of white blood cell that is an essential part of the immune system that fights disease. However, T cells are well regulated and have "off" signals. After a short period of time, these signals cause T cells to turn off, which, in most cases, is necessary to prevent them from damaging the body. However, the problem with cancer is that by the time it is detected by the body, it can be too large for T cells to eradicate. The T cells attack the cancer but turn off before they are fully effective. Immune checkpoint therapy blocks the "off" switch so the T cells can continue their work in a specified, targeted manner to eliminate the cancer. The T cell response also adapts and can accommodate tumor heterogeneity as well as respond to changes in recurring tumors. Finally, once the body learns to fight the cancer more effectively, it will *remember* and be able to do so long after the treatment has ended (Sharma & Allison, 2015). This generates immune memory (Brodsky, 2018) and allows the body to continue its work in healing itself.

Metaphorically the goal in psychotherapy, especially for patients with a history of trauma, is to provide a type of metaphorical immune therapy:

to give the patient the ability to identify a trauma trigger (metaphorically a "cancer cell") and continue to maintain vigilance in not over-reacting (not let the "cancer cells" proliferate). Further, therapy helps "kill off" the trauma trigger in a targeted manner, as the patient confronts old dysfunctional patterns and develops new patterns. Therapy also enhances the ability to adapt as trauma triggers may change over time. These factors all can increase self-regulation and lessen the trauma response.

How imagination affects biology

The imagination can trigger bodily healing. The placebo effect creates beneficial results based on the patient's response to the treatment, not on the biological action of the treatment. If one *imagines* a treatment will help, it frequently will have a healing effect. For example, a Band-Aid with a picture of Elmo might work better than a plain Band-Aid for a young child. Although estimates vary, Esther Sternberg (2009) reports that the placebo effect accounts for about one-third of the therapeutic benefit of any given medicine.

A possible explanation is placebos create positive expectations, which change the appraisal of a situation and then shape sensory and emotional processing. In pain patients, expectations that a treatment will be beneficial cause changes in the prefrontal cortex that decrease the brain's response to painful stimulation, therefore reducing the patient's experience of pain (Wagner, 2005). These pain pathways share common circuitry with other diseases, such as depression and Parkinson's.

The work of Raul de la Fuente-Fernández and Stoessl (2002) provides evidence for a placebo effect in patients with Parkinson's disease (PD). When PD patients are given a placebo, their dopamine system is activated and a substantial amount of endogenous dopamine is released. This activates the predominate pathway that is damaged in Parkinson's. The magnitude of the response is comparable to therapeutic doses of levodopa, a treatment for Parkinson's. The authors conclude that for some PD patients, most of the benefit obtained from an active drug might be based on the placebo effect.[8] They hypothesize that the dopamine release was due to an expectation of reward – in this case, a therapeutic effect. All patients were familiar with the effect of an active drug, such as levodopa, and this previous experience may have enhanced their expectations. Placebo effects are reported for many other illnesses, including alcoholism, irritable bowel syndrome, and panic and anxiety disorders. Improvements have been reported after sham surgeries for Parkinson's disease, heart disease and arthritic knee pain.

In an elegant experiment involving the placebo response, Fabrizio Benedetti et al. (2003) studied four different conditions – pain, anxiety, Parkinsonism and heart rate – under two situations: some subjects were treated openly with drugs appropriate to their condition and the others were given a hidden infusion of the *same* drugs. The openly treated group responded significantly more to the medications than the group that did not know they were being treated. Daniel Moerman and Anne Harrington (2005) suggest that it was because only the first group had the opportunity to make meaning out of the treatment.

Objecting to identifying this phenomenon as the "placebo response," Moerman and colleagues (Moerman, 2000, 2010; Moerman & Jonas, 2002) have long advocated substituting a broader concept, the "meaning response," defined as the "psychological and physiological effects of meaning in the treatment of illness" (Moerman, 2000, p. 52). According to Moerman, the placebo response is too narrow a term. The efficacy in the placebo response is not in the placebo itself but in the meaning attributed to it, emerging in part from the doctor/patient relationship and the patient's faith in the doctor's abilities (Moerman, 2000, 2010). The effect of an active drug can be enhanced by a trusted physician showing enthusiasm for the drug and displaying medical competence. Conversely, as physicians change their view of particular drugs, the effectiveness of the drugs change. Studies have suggested that when new drugs come onto the market with much excitement and advertising, physicians lose their enthusiasm for the older drugs, and these drugs in turn become less effective (Moerman & Harrington, 2005). Related, Moerman suggests that many symbolically meaningful acts occur during treatment, such as taking a history, physical examination, repeated blood pressure readings, receiving a diagnosis, and that these can have positive meaning to a patient and contribute to healing (Moerman, 2000, 2010).

Moving to the big picture: evolution

Is evolution "creative"?

The imagination of the body, including the highly complex processes of neuroplasticity, the immune response and the placebo effect, could not exist without the forces of evolution. It has succeeded in generating the myriad unique and adaptive forms of life that have lived and died on our earth for hundreds of millions of years, including humans with the ability to learn and heal. A step-by-step process, evolution is a relentless, unthinking force that creates gradual improvement in the characteristics of biological populations over successive generations by cumulative selection.

These characteristics are the expressions of genes that are passed on from parent to offspring during reproduction. Meiosis and fertilization provide enormous variation for evolution to succeed. In cumulative selection, the end product of one generation is the starting point for the next. Entities reproduce and evolve; better, more successful forms emerge. This chapter will consider whether evolution itself can be considered a creative process. If so, what can therapists learn from this force to develop more effective psychotherapy?

Revisiting an idea that was prevalent prior to the Romantic era, before 1800, Bosnak (2018) discusses the concept of "creative genius." In this view, genius is not associated with an individual; rather, it is in the material. Michelangelo said that David was in the stone. He just had to carve away the excess to reveal it. Mozart thought he received his music; he didn't "create" it. Creative genius is a force or a spirit, and we must be struck by it.

Further genius is cold, brutal and inhumane. It simply wants to manifest itself; it is up to us to receive it (Bosnak, 2018). From this perspective, *evolution is the genius*, a cold, relentless force, demanding to manifest itself. We, in various guises and forms, craft and shape our wares out of the material of evolution. As biologists, psychotherapists, writers or moviemakers, we work with the results of evolution in primary, secondary and tertiary ways.

To understand evolution, physician and Pulitzer Prize-winning author Siddhartha Mukherjee stresses the importance of understanding the nature of inheritance: "Heredity was the yin to evolution's yang" (Mukherjee, 2016. p. 66). For evolution to occur, both variation and stability are necessary. Without variation – the possibility of deep genetic diversity – an organism could lose the ability to survive in changing circumstances. For example, a finch with a wider than average beak might survive more easily in a famine because it can gather food more efficiently. Then these naturally occurring variations must be stable and able to be passed on – fixing the variation for generations to come (Mukherjee, 2016). The nature of inheritance and the giant forces of evolution go hand in hand.

With the exception of identical twins, no two children of the same parents are genetically the same. This is because before fertilization, several types of randomizing genetic reassortments happen during meiosis in the creation of the gamete (in humans, the sperm or egg). One startling example of this is called random orientation of homologous pairs, in which each sperm or egg acquires a random mixture of maternal and paternal chromosomes (Alberts et al., 2002). As background, each parent germ cell (specialized cells that are the precursors of gametes) has 23 homologous or similar pairs of chromosomes, totaling 46. Every homologous pair has one chromosome from the father and one from the mother. Each sperm or egg has 23 chromosomes, taking one chromosome from each of the 23 homologous pairs.

The randomization process occurs as follows: each of the 23 homologous pairs line up opposite each other to create the gamete. In doing so, they "shuffle" randomly, that is, the chromosome from the father can be on the right or the left and the same for the mother. Next, when they split vertically to create the 23-chromosome sperm or egg, there are multiple possibilities. A particular sperm may randomly have 14 of chromosomes from the mother and 9 from the father, while another may have 20 from the father and only 3 from the mother and so on, creating genetic variation (Griffiths et al., 2005; Gilbert, 2014). This process can create 2^{23} or over 8 million different possibilities or assortments. The same is true for the egg. This makes 8 million × 8 million totaling 64 trillion possible combinations during fertilization.[9] Yet this seemingly endless variation is within the context of stability because every chromosome is taken from one of the parents.

In certain cases, this enormous variation contributes to the possibility of "choice" or genetic preference at the moment of fertilization. Conventional wisdom is that fertilization is random or that the fastest sperm fertilizes the egg. Recent research (Arnold, 2017; Nadeau, 2017) hypothesizes that, in some cases, other factors may play a role. Although not yet well understood, possibly the egg could attract a sperm with specific genes and vice versa. This causes certain unions to be more probable than others, in some cases possibly avoiding the inheritance of mutant genes. For example, one factor suggested is the female immune system may play a role in sperm selection. The mechanisms that might cause this nonrandom fertilization are not yet clear, and additional research is needed to examine how the interaction of the sperm and egg can influence fertilization.

A further example of biological imagination is that DNA can repair itself "creatively." DNA repair is crucial; failure to do so increases the likelihood of developing tumors and other diseases. One example is a process called homologous recombination. When DNA is damaged by a mutagen, such as X-rays, the part that is damaged can be recopied from its twin chromosome and inserted in place of the damaged part – that is, a part on the maternal chromosome can be copied to repair the analogous part on the paternal chromosome. Proteins coordinate the process, helping the gene correct itself by "... guiding the damaged strand to the intact gene, copying and correcting the lost information, and stitching the breaks together ...." (Mukherjee, 2016, p. 182). In this way, the undamaged strand transfers the needed information to the damaged strand. These processes again demonstrate Kaag's notion of the biological basis of imagination, how our body is capable of creating new variations within existing structures and can meet unforeseen circumstances and spontaneously repair itself.

Artificial intelligence

In viewing the principles of evolution as possible tools for insight into creativity and imagination, I focus on the work of design engineers (French, 1994) and computer scientists (Bentley & Corne, 2002), who truly appreciate the amazingly creative end products of evolutionary forces. Computer scientists are using algorithms based on principles of evolution to produce impressive works in art, music, product design and architecture.

Investigators of artificial intelligence, Peter Bentley and David Corne (2002) argue that evolution exhibits some of the properties of creativity. A master of design, evolution's end products resemble creative solutions, such as the chemical factories inside our cells or the very complicated organization of our brain. Evolution has created an organism only 3 mm long that flies, has vision, can sustain itself by converting chemicals into energy and is even able to reproduce itself (a fly) – while human technology cannot yet do that. Many modern inventions are taken directly from nature, for example, the cross-sectional shape of aircraft wings from birds and Velcro from certain types of "sticky" seeds (Bentley & Corne, 2002). The inventors of these products were visionaries who could use the "genius" of evolution to create products for our use.

The principles of natural selection have been applied to computers, endowing them with skills that resemble creativity (Bentley, 1999; Bentley & Corne, 2002). Through a process called evolutionary design, the computer is programmed to evolve designs and produce creative products in many fields, harnessing the power of evolution for nonliving designs.[10] The evolutionary algorithm is guided to find the best solution to a problem according to a fitness function, that is, how well the solution fits the program objective, such as creating an airplane with more legroom.

However, this is an emergent process and not explicitly stated in the algorithm (Bentley, 1999). The researchers that write the program cannot predict the results of a program until it runs (Lehman et al., 2018). The researchers are frequently surprised by the results, just as our patients can surprise us and develop in ways not previously imagined.

To explain the process, Bentley and Corne (2002) discuss the foundational concept of "search" in artificial intelligence, the long journey through an immense space of possibilities in search of something suitable. Based on evolutionary principles, evolutionary search is a rapidly growing, efficient and creative subset of search algorithms. Instead of working with one solution at a time, these algorithms consider large population of solutions at once and perform search operations by mimicking the process of natural selection, that is, by evolving solutions to problems. From the large population of solutions, the computer allows better solutions to "reproduce" or have "children," while worse solutions die. The "children" inherit their "parents'" characteristics with small variations. This continues, and after a number of generations, if successful, the computer will have satisfied the fitness function. This is an automatic generation of innovation, much like natural evolution itself.

One of the benefits of this type of algorithm is that it is not biased in the beginning; rather it is open to any and all possibilities. Then through an emergent process, the problem gradually gets solved, similar to the work of the psychotherapist. Alluding to Bion, the therapist enters the session without memory or desire, that is, he entertains the large collection of possibilities at once and is not biased in a particular direction. But within this open framework, the therapist guides. Ideas and feelings bubble up into consciousness. The therapeutic dyad accepts certain of these possibilities and discards others, depending on whether they "fit" with the patient, his feelings and goals. In this way, understanding evolves. This emergent process coupled with the fitness function is part of what makes psychotherapeutic work so creative. Evolutionary algorithms have captured this process as well.

A researcher specializing in genetic algorithms, a type of evolutionary algorithm that most resembles natural selection, David Goldberg (1999) makes interesting connections between evolutionary processes, human innovation and his work in genetic algorithms. He cites two different facets of human innovation: (1) the *improvement type* that involves selection and mutation and (2) the *cross-fertilizing type* that involves selection and recombination. Both types of innovation can be applied to genetic algorithms.

In human behavior, we see the improvement type in terms of the quest for continual improvement in finding better and better solutions, such as the Japanese concept of kaizen, an approach to creating continuous improvement, especially in business, based on the idea that small, ongoing positive changes or variants ("mutations") can be selected to reap major improvements.

The cross-fertilizing type occurs when people take an idea in one context and juxtapose it with an idea in another, speculating that the combination might be better than either idea taken individually. Goldberg (1999, p. 108) quotes the French mathematician Jacques Hadamard, "Indeed, it is obvious that invention or discovery, be it in mathematics or anywhere else, takes place by combining ideas." This is somewhat analogous to the genetic variation created by chromosomes recombining in novel ways to create variation. Regarding genetic algorithms, the cross-fertilization process helps translate the more local findings of gradual improvement, that is, improvement in one specific area, and applies them more broadly, what Goldberg (1999, p. 108) terms "intelligent jumping." Goldberg focuses on the cross-fertilizing type.

This volume discusses both types of innovation in relation to psychotherapy: (1) the gradual improvement we see in work with a patient that can lead to an "aha" moment that creates seemingly sudden change and (2) the cross-fertilization type, in this volume's emphasis on dreamwork and interdisciplinary approaches. The next chapter, Chapter 6, explores the many odd and unique combinations of images in dreamwork and how to cross-fertilize them to create change. Chapter 8 takes the many gradual improvements in the field of psychotherapy and juxtaposes them with concepts in other fields to search for innovative solutions.

What's psychotherapy got to do with it?

The scourge of the repetition compulsion, one of the main causes of psychopathology, is that the same pattern is repeated over and over, with no evolution. For new behaviors to emerge in patients mired in this compulsion, variation must be introduced. At times, the variation will come in the form of an event, either in session or in the patient's life, which helps disrupt the repetitive behavior and then psychotherapy can build on this. In a troubled or abusive marriage, it is frequently an event within the relationship. This can precipitate a "mutation" of sorts, a new slant or reconfiguration, that allows the patient to consider new possibilities.

Suddenly, victimhood is relinquished

Fifty-year-old Becky has been married to Leon for 25 years. The marriage is unhappy and Becky is aware that Leon has had multiple affairs. Ostensibly, Becky remained with Leon because of their child Sophie, now 21. However, Becky is actually mired in a repetitive enactment of bitterness and despair, a close replica of her own parents' marriage, during which both parents were unfaithful.

Becky tells her story in detail. Recently, on the first night of Passover, she and Leon are setting up a Seder for family and friends. The dining table is prepared. Although somewhat depressed, Becky has made all the customary celebratory foods. Her challah, brisket and kugel are on display. Suddenly Paul, secretly invited by Leon, arrives. Becky is shocked and angry as she immediately knows Leon invited him for revenge. Leon is aware that over 20 years ago, Becky had an affair with Paul, during which time Sophie was conceived. Paul and his family moved away shortly afterward, and Sophie is not aware that Paul is her biological father.

Becky senses that tonight Leon is going to expose the identity of Sophie's real father. Becky and Paul have seen each other sporadically over the years and just recently spent a night together at a nearby motel. Unbeknownst to Becky, Leon accidentally found a receipt from that night. Leon begins to taunt:

> So Paul, have you seen the new Thunderbird Motel, across from the Home Depot? Huh, have you Paul? Your scandal didn't stop 20 years ago like Becky told me. Yeah, Paul, I found the Thunderbird Motel receipt for the two of you from last week.

To retort, Becky jumps up and turns to Leon, "Well, you weren't perfect either. There were women. But my mistake with Paul? He's (Leon) hated me ever since." Becky continues to Sophie:

> You know the first time the word hate comes up in the Bible –it's not for the enemies of Israel – it's a man for his wife – Jacob hated his wife, Leah. He wanted her sister, and you know who your father wants – those other women!

Turning to Paul, Becky says:

> So, you, Paul, would talk to me. You would listen to me. Leon never did. You know I wished he took a lesson from our father Abraham in the Bible. Abraham would give his beautiful wife Sarah – he called her his "sister" – to foreign kings, so they wouldn't fight him for her. I wish Leon gave me to you. When I was with you – this was the first time I felt love. And when I became pregnant, I was thrilled. You know I couldn't have children with Leon. I wanted to leave him.

Becky's wish for change, which has been simmering for a long time, suddenly erupts. The arrival of Paul sparks a vitality and productive anger in Becky that creates enough agency for her to tell Sophie about her biological father and finally, to end the marriage. Ironically, at this point, Leon tries to reconcile. Becky screams at him that it's too late, that she has had a 25-year sentence with him. At the end of the evening, Becky triumphantly says to Sophie:

> You and me. Before I was gonna just push my food in everyone's face. 'Here! Take my life!' Like he (Leon) has all these years. But now, some wine and enjoy before the guests arrive. Come, my first night of freedom.

This is where psychotherapy could help Becky build on her "aha" moment, her new agency and courage. However, Becky is not a real patient. She is a character in my play "Abba's Surprise." (Abba is Hebrew for father.) This play is based on my work with many people trapped in relationships. The same dysfunctional patterns are repeatedly reenacted until something sparks a change, and they can forge the agency to build on it. In real life, Becky would need therapeutic support to solidify relinquishing the "victim" stance. She needs to become aware of how she has been enacting aspects of her parents' marriage. The Seder night, however, is the beginning of the transformation.

Expanding the imagination

The writings of Bentley and Corne provided some "supervision" for me with my patient Emma, an example of cross-fertilization, as I played with applying the workings of evolutionary design to psychotherapy.

A 65-year-old college professor in educational psychology and communications, Emma is very anxious and uncertain about retirement. She is required to retire soon and is fearful of becoming depressed. Without her work, she feels unable to structure a meaningful life for herself. We have been approaching this psychotherapeutically for some time, and she still could not "conceive" of what direction to take. I had not been able to help her dissolve old patterns of avoidance (unwire old connections) and generate new ones moving toward solutions (wire new connections).

Reflecting on this, I decided to vary my approach and guide more, similar to what the AI scientists do in evolutionary design. Perhaps she and I could generate a large population of possibilities concerning activities in retirement, and between sessions, she can put them to her own fitness test. Will this activity/approach/perspective be meaningful and contribute to a satisfying retirement?

I suggest an experiment to Emma. Explaining I have been reading about evolutionary design, I propose we adapt some of the strategies. We can generate multiple possibilities together, and she can try them out between sessions. When she works through the first series of ideas, she picks several of the best. Then she develops these more fully and from that generates several more. This continues until she finds several really good solutions. This may help her "learn," in Kandel's sense, both to develop a new approach to solving problems and to find some specific long-term solutions.

After we talk through pitfalls, she becomes enthusiastic, acknowledging, "This will counter my tendency to shoot down every idea, and I like it. It seems like a game." This approach is also familiar to her, as she enjoys designing strategies for her students. Then right after she says she likes the approach, she spontaneously has a new idea and comments, "I'm tired of working with college students. I want to get down on the floor with young kids and have some fun. I could develop games based on neuroscience. This would be a dream!"

She has had a growing interest in neuroscience and how the brain learns. She wants to develop games for elementary age children that teach specific skills in language arts and math as well as adapt to the child's learning style to help him or her become an independent learner. Several sessions later, she expands the idea, "I can also teach parents how to use the games with children who are struggling."

Emma allowed an idea to pop up, breaking the stalemate of not knowing. I comment on this, and she associates to her mother, "I had to be a good girl. I could never cause disruption. She never let me be angry." When I say how hard this must have been, she replies, "Perhaps, but I learned to suppress, suppress everything. Really, after a while I stopped knowing what I felt."

"So, she succeeded but you suffered," I say.

Emma: "To tell you the truth I didn't know. I idolized her."

LD: "Until now, when you need to see the nuances, some good, some bad."

These fixed ideas that Emma had – she should never be angry, especially never criticize her mother – prevented her from flexibly imagining her next steps.

Several weeks later, the experiment starts to break down and she stops exploring. When I press her for what is blocking her, she bursts out, "But I'm so scared. Can't you see?" In fact, it *is* hard for me to see because she is well spoken and doesn't show fear easily and also perhaps because of my ambition for her. I acknowledge I do not fully see and ask her to say more.

Emma: "I'm afraid I won't succeed. That I will let you down. That I can't do it. It seems so easy for you. I feel ashamed."

Apparently, like her, I too must look calm and collected. I tell her, however, that I am also afraid and as an example, refer to my multiple anxieties about writing this book. We speak about fear as natural when attempting something new. The tricky part is how to press past the fear. She asks me how I do it. I have to think for a moment. Then I give the best answer I can, "My curiosity is what does it. If I am really excited about a project, my curiosity drives me to keep working and overrides my fear." This cycle of forward movement and stalemate continues, as Emma struggles to break long-standing patterns of fear and avoidance.

The work of Bentley and Corne gave us the push, which at first stimulated ideas and then allowed the resistance to emerge more clearly and therefore become easier to explore. Harkening back to evolution, resistance to change may be universal as we need both stability (which resistance serves) as well as variation for evolutionary change to be productive. This example of using principles of AI is given only to suggest how therapists can gather ideas from other fields, not that the specific approach of using AI would work with other patients. Each patient needs a metaphor crafted for him or her.

To conclude

Providing variation to our thinking, exploring the adjacent field of biology makes it possible to understand imagination and psychotherapy more deeply. The imaginative activity we witness in life exists at the cellular level. Out of conscious awareness and using a mixture of stability and novelty, the body spontaneously meets unexpected circumstances in acts of adaptive imagination.

These biological processes suggest direction for the therapist. Referring back to the neuronal concept of reentry, the dyad can strive to become more improvisational, like members of jazz ensemble, as they work together to help the patient refine existing patterns and develop new ones. The discussion about the placebo effect reminds the therapist of the importance of developing the most meaningful therapeutic alliance she can so the patient develops faith and trust in the treatment. Finally, just as immunotherapy helps the body remember to fight cancer long after the treatment ends, the clinician strives to do the same so that after termination, the patient continues to adapt and benefit.

Referencing evolution, the therapist can ask herself if the patient is evolving. Dawkins (1996) emphasizes the importance of gradual, step-by-step change in evolution, which has much better chance of success than large quick random changes. If a child mutates very significantly from its parent – that is a large, quick change – he or she is unlikely to survive. To give an everyday analogy, if a patient makes a small change, say cleans up a very small section of his chronically disorganized desk, this is significant, and further change may be forthcoming. The likelihood of a large and abrupt change achieving sustainable organization is slim. However, at other times, either the patient or the therapist can have an "aha" moment where change does seem sudden (Domash, 2010). An idea or memory can erupt and spark a turning point. However, frequently these insights have actually emerged from prior unconscious work in therapy.

The processes of evolution and the workings of genes and chromosomes elucidate principles of creativity. While it is not clear whether one can call the blind force of evolution creative, the results of the process surely are. Consider the interesting process of exaptation, when structures evolved for one use are opportunistically or "inventively" adapted for other purposes (Gould & Vrba, 1982; Lehman et al., 2018). A leading theory is that feathers first evolved in dinosaurs for temperature regulation (Kundŕat, 2004) and were later exapted for flight in birds. This reminds us of the need for inventiveness in everyday life and how one might take advantage of what is already in place, either emotionally or physically.

Evolution needs variation to do its work. Beginning with the formation of the sperm or the egg, millions of variations are possible in conception. This gives a huge population of novel possibilities, creating diversity and choice for the best solution. For the therapeutic dyad to move forward, variation is also needed. Programs such as the study of Embodied Imagination is but one of myriad possibilities for therapists to broaden their repertoire in order to help stimulate the imagination of the patient.

While patients need to develop mental flexibility to produce variations in perspective and behavior, they also must remain continuous with the past. Edelman's "remembered present" – the past mingled with the present – defines human consciousness and occupies the therapeutic dyad. Therapist and patient refine memories of the past and integrate them with the present as they work toward change. This repairs states of emotional brokenness and dysregulation while preserving the continuity of the self.

For psychodynamic therapists, understanding patients is an evolving, emergent process, echoing the forces of evolution. The therapist listens carefully and formulates with the patient, then listens again and formulates a little better. Gradually, answers emerge as the therapist helps the patient evolve and find the best ("fittest") solutions for interacting with her world.

Notes

1 DNA (deoxyribonucleic acid) is the carrier of genetic information. It not only contains all the hereditary information necessary to build and maintain an organism but also serves as the primary unit of heredity. Whenever organisms reproduce, they pass along a portion of their DNA, ensuring both continuity and slight changes that create diversity in the next generation (https://www.nature.com/scitable/topicpage/introduction-what-is-dna-6579978/).

2 However, while many of these biological processes happen regardless of our state of mind, anxiety and stress can interfere with the "biological imagination," just as anxiety and stress can stifle the psychological imagination. In a review article, Sheldon Cohen et al. (2007) report established associations between psychological stress and disease, particularly for depression, cardiovascular disease and HIV/AIDS. Evidence for the role of stress is also beginning to emerge in upper respiratory tract infections, asthma, herpes viral infections, autoimmune diseases and wound healing.

3 A gene is a hereditary unit passed from parent to offspring consisting of a sequence of DNA. Some viruses, store genetic information in RNA. The entire

set of genetic instructions carried by an organism (termed a genome) comprises approximately 24,000 protein-coding genes (International Human Genome Sequencing Consortium, 2004) that provide the instructions to build, repair and maintain our body and mind. However, estimates of the total number vary. The number may be much higher, depending on how a gene is defined (Salzberg, 2018). The definition of a gene is evolving as new information becomes available.

4 A chromosome is a very long, single DNA helix consisting of thousands of genes. Twenty-three pairs of chromosomes are inherited from parents (46 in total). One chromosome from each of the 23 pairs comes from each parent.

5 The somatosensory cortex is an area of the brain that processes sensory input from the body and helps interpret information regarding temperature, pressure, pain and touch as well as the position of the body in space. Neurons from different parts of the body receive environmental stimuli and send their information to the somatosensory cortex for processing. Specific parts of the cortex are associated with specific areas of the body. If the area of the brain that represents the left thumb is stimulated, the person will feel sensations in that finger (https://www.alleydog.com/glossary/definition.php?term=Somatosensory+Cortex).

6 While most of the research is in the premotor area, mirror neurons in monkeys have also been found in the primary motor cortex and the parietal lobe.

7 According to Kilner and Lemon (2013), it is difficult to measure and interpret mirror neuron activity in humans. The techniques for investigating these in monkeys are too invasive for human studies. It is important to use caution when comparing results from human and monkey studies on mirror neuron activity.

8 Cynthia McRae et al. (2004) report a dramatic example in a study using sham surgery to determine the effectiveness of transplants of embryonic dopamine neurons into the brains of persons with advanced Parkinson's disease. In the study, all 39 subjects had four holes drilled in their skulls under local anesthesia. Half of them actually got the transplants, while the other half received sham surgery (no treatment other than having holes drilled). The study maintained the double-blind phase, that is, patients continued not to know which surgery they had, for one year after the surgery. Patients in the sham surgery group were able to get the actual surgery after the double-blind was lifted.

McRae et al. did a follow-up study at one year and found that, overall, patients who thought they had the actual surgery reported a better quality of life – regarding not only emotional and social functioning but motor functioning as well – than patients who thought they received sham surgery, regardless of which surgery they received. The medical staff confirmed the physical improvements. The placebo effect in this study was very strong. Although sham surgery is controversial and raises ethical concerns, the researchers in this study determined that the potential benefits outweighed the ethical concerns.

9 The actual number is greater than this due to another type of random reassortment during meiosis called recombination or crossing over, during which genetic information is swapped between homologous chromosomes in the parent germ cell. DNA from the maternal chromosome can exchange positions with DNA from the paternal chromosome – generating a gene hybrid of maternal and paternal genes. This swapping of genetic information occurs at places on the chromosome that do not break genetic information and disrupt development, an example of the billions of years of evolution that have optimized opportunities for successful variation to happen. This process occurs earlier in the meiosis process than the random orientation of homologous pairs, described in the text (https://bodell.mtchs.org/OnlineBio/BIOCD/text/chapter9/concept9.6.html).

10 Bentley (1999) measured the results of music produced by computer (using evolutionary design) with the Turing test, reasoning that if people cannot

distinguish between the results of the computer and the results of human creativity, then the results of the computer could be considered creative. He describes an experiment in which music was played to three groups. The first two groups were art and design Master's students and staff and the third group were computer scientists. The first minute of three songs were played, and after having listened to all three, the audiences were asked which song they thought had been evolved by a computer. The first two groups could not tell the difference between computer-produced music and man-made music. Only the third group, comprised of computer scientists, could. Bentley concluded it is possible for the results of evolutionary design to be considered creative, at least for some people.

References

Alberts, B., Johnson, A., Lewis, J., Raff, M., Roberts, K. & Walter, P. (2002). *Molecular biology of the cell*, Fourth edition. New York: Garland Science.

Arnold, C. (November 15, 2017). Choosy eggs may pick sperm for their genes, defying Mendel's Law. *Quanta Magazine*. Online. https://www.quantamagazine.org/choosy-eggs-may-pick-sperm-for-their-genes-defying-mendels-law-20171115/

Benedetti, F., Maggi, G., Lopiano, L., Lanotte, M., Rainero, I., Vighetti, S. & Pollo, A. (2003). Open versus hidden medical treatments: The patient's knowledge about a therapy affects the therapy outcome. *Prevention & Treatment,* 6 (1): Article 1a: no pagination specified. http://dx.doi.org/10.1037/1522-3736.6.1.61a

Bentley, P.J. (1999). Is evolution creative? In P.J. Bentley and D.W. Corne (Eds.), *Proceedings of the AISB'99 Symposium on Creative Evolutionary Systems (CES)* (pp. 28–34), Society for the Study of Artificial Intelligence and Stimulation of Behaviour.

Bentley, P.J. & Corne, D.W. (2002). An introduction to creative evolutionary systems. In P.J. Bentley and D.W. Corne (Eds.), *Creative evolutionary systems* (pp. 1–75). San Diego. CA: Academic Press.

Bosnak, R. (2018). *Inviting creative genius into your life.* Webinar, Jung Platform. February 1, 2018–June 28, 2018.

Brodsky, A.N. (2018). Dr. James P. Allison, CRI Scientific Director, Awarded 2018 Nobel Prize along with Dr. Tasuku Honjo. cancerresearch.org/blog/October-2018. https://www.cancerresearch.org/blog/october-2018/james-allison-et-al-2018-nobel-prize-physio-med

Cohen, S., Janicki-Deverts, D. & Miller, G.E. (2007). Psychological stress and disease. *Journal of the American Medical Association*, 298(14):1685–1687.

Dawkins, R. (1996). *The blind watchmaker: Why the evidence of evolution reveals a universe without design*. New York: W.W. Norton.

Doidge, N. (2007). *The brain that changes itself: Stories of personal triumph from the frontiers of brain science*. New York: Penguin Books.

Doidge, N. (2015). *The brain's way of healing: Remarkable discoveries and recoveries from the frontiers of neuroplasticity*. New York: Penguin Books.

Domash, L. (2010). Unconscious freedom and the insight of the analyst: Exploring neuropsychological processes underlying 'aha' moments. *Journal of The American Academy of Psychoanalysis and Dynamic Psychiatry*, 38:315–339.

Edelman, G. (1987). *Neural Darwinism: The theory of neuronal group selection.* New York: Basic Books.

Edelman, G. (1999). Building a picture of the brain. *Annals of the New York Academy of Science*, 882(1):68–89.

Edelman, G. & Tononi, G. (2000). *A universe of consciousness: How matter becomes imagination*. Cambridge, MA: Perseus Books.

Feldman, D.E. & Brecht, M. (2005). Map plasticity in somatosensory cortex. *Science*, 310:810–815.

Fox, J. (1984). The brain's dynamic way of keeping in touch. *Science*, 225:820.

French, M.J. (1994). *Invention and evolution: Design in nature and Engineering*, Second edition. Cambridge, UK: Cambridge University Press.

Freud, S. (1895). Project for a scientific psychology. *Standard Edition*, 1:281–397.

de la Fuente-Fernández, R. & Stoessl, A.J. (2002). The placebo effect in Parkinson's disease. *Trends in Neuroscience*, 25(6):302–306.

Gallese, V. (1996). Action recognition in the premotor cortex. *Brain*, 119:593–609.

Gallese, V., Eagle, M.N. & Migone, P. (2007). Intentional attunement: Mirror neurons and the neural underpinnings of interpersonal relations. *Journal of the American Psychoanalytic Association*, 55(1):131–176.

Gilbert, S.F. (2014). *Developmental Biology*. Sunderland, MA: Sinauer Associates, Inc.

Goldberg, D. (1999). The race, the hurdle, and the sweet spot: Lessons from genetic algorithms for the automation of design innovation and creativity. In P.J. Bentley (Ed.), *Evolutionary design by computers* (pp. 105–118). San Francisco, CA: Morgan Kaufmann.

Gould, S.J. & Vrba, E.S. (1982). Exaptation – A missing term in the science of form. *Paleobiology*, 8(1):4–15.

Griffiths, J.F., Gelbart, W.M., Lewontin, R.C., Wessler, S.R., Suzuki, D.T. & Miller, J.H. (2005). *Introduction to genetic analysis*. New York: W.H. Freeman.

Hebb, D. (1949). *The organization of behavior: A neuropsychological theory*. New York: John Wiley.

International Human Genome Sequencing Consortium. (2004). Finishing the euchromatic sequence of the human genome. *Nature*, 431(7011):931–945.

Jarrett, C. (December 13, 2013). A calm look at the most hyped concept in neuroscience – Mirror neurons. *Wired*, Science. https://www.wired.com/2013/12/a-calm-look-at-the-most-hyped-concept-in-neuroscience-mirror-neurons/

Kaag, J. (2008). The neurological dynamics of the imagination. *Phenomenology and the Cognitive Sciences*, 8:183–204.

Kaag, J. (2014). *Thinking through the imagination: Aesthetics in human cognition*. New York: Fordham University Press.

Kandel, E.R. (1998). A new intellectual framework for psychiatry. *American Journal of Psychiatry*, 155(4):457–469.

Kilner, J.M. & Lemon, R.N. (2013). What we currently know about mirror neurons. *Current Biology*, 23(23):R1057–R1062.

Kundŕat, M. (2004). When did theropods become feathered? – Evidence for pre-Archaeopteryx feathery appendages. *Journal of Experimental Zoology Part B: Molecular and Developmental Evolution*, 302(4):355–364.

Lehman, J., Clune, J. Misevic, D., Adami, C., Altenberg, L., Beaulieu, J., Bentley, P.J., Bernard, S., Beslon, G., Bryson, D.M., Chrabaszcz, P., Cheney, N., Cully, A., Doncieux, S., Dyer, F.C., Ellefsen, K.O., Feldt, R., Fischer, S., Forrest, S., Frénoy, A.,

Gagné, C., LeGoff, L., Grabowski, L.M., Hodjat, B., Hutter, F., et al. (28 additional authors not shown) (2018). The surprising creativity of digital evolution: A collection of anecdotes from the evolutionary computation and artificial life research communities. arXiv Labs, Cornell University. arXiv:1803.03453v3 [cs.NE].

Mason, J.M. (Trans. and Ed.) (1985). *The complete letters of Sigmund Freud to Wilhelm Fliess.* Cambridge: MA: Harvard University Press.

McRae, C., Chernin, E., Yamazaki, T.G., Diem, G., Vo, A.H., Russell, D., Ellgring, J.H., Fahn, S., Greene, P., Dillon, S., Winfield, H., Bjugstad, K.B. & Freed, C.R. (2004). Effects of perceived treatment on quality of life and medical outcomes in a double-blind placebo surgery trial. *Archives of General Psychiatry*, 61:412–420.

Moerman, D.E. (2000). Cultural variations in the placebo effect: ulcers, anxiety, and blood pressure. *Medical Anthropology Quarterly*, 14:1–22.

Moerman, D.E. (2010). *Meaning, medicine, and the "placebo effect."* Cambridge: Cambridge University Press.

Moerman, D.E., & Harrington, A. (2005). Making space for the placebo effect in pain medicine. *Seminars in Pain Medicine*, 3(1):2–6.

Moerman, D.E. & Jonas, W.B. (2002). Deconstructing the placebo effect and finding the meaning response. *Annals of Internal Medicine*, 136(6):471–476.

Mukherjee, S. (2016). *The gene: An intimate history.* New York: Scribner.

Nadeau, J.H. (October 1, 2017). Do Gametes Woo? Evidence for their nonrandom union at fertilization. *Genetics*, 207(2):369–387.

Ringstrom, P. (2001). Cultivating the improvisational in psychoanalytic treatment. *Psychoanalytic Dialogues*, 11(5):727–754.

Rizzolatti, G. & Craighero, L. (2004). The mirror-neuron system. *Annual Review of Neuroscience*, 27:169–192.

Salzberg, S. (2018). Open questions: How many genes do we have? *BMC Biology*, 16:94.

Sharma, P. & Allison, J. (2015). Immune checkpoint targeting in cancer therapy: Toward combination strategies with curative potential. *Cell*, 161(2):205–214.

Sternberg, E. (2009). Can believing make you well? In S. Aizenstat & R. Bosnak (Eds.), *Imagination and medicine: The future of healing in an age of neuroscience* (pp. 87–106). New Orleans, LA: Spring Journal Books.

Umiltà, M., Kohler, E., Gallese V., Fogassi, L., Fadiga, L., Keysers, C. & Rizzolatti, G. (2001). I know what you are doing: A neurophysiological study. *Neuron*, 31:155–165.

Vaughn, S.C. (1997). *The talking cure: The science behind psychotherapy.* New York: Grosset/Putnam.

Wagner, T. (2005). The neural bases of placebo effects in pain. *Current Directions in Psychological Science*, 14(4):175–179.

Chapter 6

Transformative dreamwork

Embodied Imagination[1]

The dream is an involuntary act of poetry.
Jean Paul Richter (quoted in Darwin, 1879/2004, p. 95)

I remember the first time I heard the Jungian psychoanalyst Robert Bosnak (1996, 1998, 2008) speak about his dream technique. In a small, warmly lit auditorium of a psychoanalytic institute in NYC, he gave a live demonstration of his approach. Bosnak began by asking the audience for a volunteer to tell a dream. He eased the volunteer into a semi-hypnotic state and the audience as well. We followed him and his resonant, confident voice as he encouraged the volunteer to tell the dream and proceed to work it according to his startlingly fresh method, Embodied Imagination (EI). I was intrigued. After taking several more weekend workshops, I decided to enter a three-year intensive training program at the LA Embodied Imagination Institute and have found this method transformative both for my patients and myself.

EI is specifically designed to expand and enhance the imagination. In the Jungian tradition, the approach works intensively with images in the dream, creating new networks and embodied states. In addition to its use with patients, this powerful technique is also used with actors, directors, writers, scientists and artists to solve artistic and scientific problems. Its goal is to help the dreamer leave what Bosnak calls his "habitual consciousness," his usual way of seeing the world, and form new approaches and perspectives. This is the essence of imagination: to stretch to see something new and not simply reproduce what one already knows.

Usual psychoanalytic dreamwork relies on the associations of the dreamer to create meaning, which is interpreted verbally. However, EI cautions that the meaning given in dream interpretation may be purely a cultural phenomenon. One culture sees the images as ancestors, another as spirits. Our culture frequently views the images as different or dissociated parts of the self, an approach originating with Jung who saw each element of the dream as an aspect of the self.

In EI there is little explicit discussion of meaning; rather, it works at an implicit level. The meaning is embedded in the images themselves and how they unconsciously work together to create new patterns, which unfold in the weeks to come after processing the dream. The dreamer is encouraged to embody the images to facilitate a "conversation" among them, with the purpose of generating new patterns and phenomena.

Objecting to the contemporary notion of imagination as the *opposite of reality*, Bosnak views the dream, which exists in a world somewhere between matter and spirit, as *real,* a quasi-physical expression of creative imagination. In the dream world, we "know" we are meeting other selves, although they disappear as soon as we wake up. Further, we can sense strong responses in our body to this quasi-physical environment. In EI, these responses are developed and amplified to help the dreamer enter the dream images in waking life to eventually create new ways of seeing and behaving.

In brief, the technique of EI is as follows: It begins with the therapist using relaxation methods to guide the patient into a state of reverie, a form of consciousness (hypnagogic) between waking and sleeping. This helps the dreamer as she recounts the dream in waking life get closer to the dreaming state and more fluidly experience different states of being. Then the therapist guides the patient to begin work on his or her dream. It is not a "waking dream" that arises out of the in-session hypnagogic state but a dream the patient has remembered and brings to the session.

During this phase of the work, the therapist helps the patient empathically embody, that is, feel in her body, selected images in her dream, usually one that is more her usual or "habitual" self (often a safe but rigid structure) and several that are "other" than how she sees herself. This defamiliarizes the familiar, a necessary ingredient to activate creativity. Then, using the several images that the patient has embodied, the therapist combines them to form a "composite," that is, a composition of the key images in the dream, which connect each state the patient has felt during the work. The patient practices (mentally reviews) the composite daily for several weeks after the session.

Rather than seeing these "other" images as fragmented or dissociated parts of the self, they are viewed as "alien intelligences" (Bosnak, 2008, p. 11), from which the dreamer can learn. This "otherness" of the image is important because, as Bosnak (2008, p. 21) writes, "Becoming infused with alien intelligences results in unexpected original flashes" that activate the imagination.

By juxtaposing the patient's familiar self with "alien intelligences," EI challenges the habitual self, which is an identification with fixed habits of consciousness. Just as we identify with our habitual consciousness, we also possess mimicry or mimesis (Taussig, 1993), which means we have the capacity, indeed, even the compulsion, to imitate others. As the dreamer imitates a "character" or image in his dream, he is pulled into the image. It comes "alive" in his body as he momentarily identifies with it. Thus, the patient empathically experiences the "alien" image as if from within, widening his imaginative resources. An actor, for example, uses this capacity to feel into and create a character very different from what she views as her usual self.

Based on Bosnak's contributions and confirmed by my personal and clinical experience and that of my colleagues, it is reasonable to hypothesize that this approach alters the repetition compulsion by accessing early memories (from the dream images), combining them in novel ways and holding them in mind simultaneously. It is possible this creates new underlying neural networks (Hebb, 1949; Kaag, 2009; Kosslyn & Moulton, 2009) and new implicit memories. By "new," Stephen Kosslyn and Samuel Moulton remind us that, for adults, this may mean modifications or recombinations of preexisting information, which produce representations or images that previously did not fully enter consciousness, that is, modifications and recombinations of preexisting information that are, nonetheless, new.

Many clinicians suggest that the key to unlocking dysfunctional behavior patterns lies in the imagination. Bromberg (2013) writes that as the capacity to transform fantasy into imagination increases, the imagined begins to feel possible. Self-states can be negotiated more smoothly, allowing the present and the future to be bridged. Less defended, the patient can entertain and actualize possibilities. Modell (2008) emphasizes that we are meant to express what is unique about ourselves: to self-actualize. This requires agency and the creation of new meanings. To do this, clinicians and patients alike need free access to an open and flexible consciousness.

The work of EI helps the dreamer reach underlying metaphoric processes, considered foundational to the imagination. Metaphor[2] is now generally accepted as a fundamental mode of cognition, not merely a figure of speech or a feature of language (Modell, 2006, 2009). Further, Modell writes, the very act of empathizing is utilizing metaphor as it plays with similarity and difference. Empathy involves an identification with the other while simultaneously maintaining one's own sense of self. Without this play of similarity/difference, one might experience a total merger with the other.

In the work of Embodied Imagination, this may be understood thus: as the patient embodies the dream image through empathic identification – that is, as she or he enters the image and feels it in the body – the patient is employing an open and fluid use of metaphor and expanding the imagination. During the work, he enters many different types of images but remains himself at the same time, experiencing a dual consciousness, a sense of similarity while maintaining difference.

Using this technique, therapists are helping the patient "dream" new capacities. Dreaming naturally combines imagery in intense, novel and incongruous ways, often with highly emotional content (Stickgold et al., 2001). Using the technique of EI, the clinician chooses images and combines them to create new patterns and possibilities. Thus, the clinician is modeling the natural process of dreaming, except she is actively deciding on the images to be combined.

Complexity theory is utilized to provide a theoretical basis for working with the composite: if we create a network of images that is neither too inert nor too chaotic and push this network to the edge of chaos, something qualitatively new is created. In this realm, which is nearly out of control but still responding to patterning, a tipping point occurs. A qualitatively different state, a "third," emerges and becomes stabilized at a more complex level than before. This is the transformational moment.

In EI, practicing the composite intensifies the connections among the complex images, accelerating change by bringing the system closer to the edge of chaos. This shores up potential fault lines and reorganizes conflicting elements into a more complex pattern. The whole system gains elasticity, resulting in a more versatile sense of self and greater ability to actualize creative potential.

Expanding the imagination of the patient

Many of our dysfunctional patterns develop from early implicit memories, creating changes in the brain's networks, resulting in lasting patterns of attachment and self-regulation (Schore, 1994, 2005; Siegel, 1999, 2007; Cozolino, 2002, 2006; Mancia, 2006; Ginot, 2007, 2015). In this context, the term "implicit memory" refers to early schemas or unconscious "knowings" about the world and ourselves. I am referring to the emotional or affective dimension of implicit memory.

Implicit memories store the early emotional and affective, at times traumatic, presymbolic and preverbal experiences of the primary mother-infant dyad (Mancia, 2006). Psychoanalyst Mauro Mancia writes they form the early, unrepressed unconscious nucleus of the self. Although formed very early, these memories can condition the affective, emotional, cognitive and sexual life of the adult. However, while these memories create lasting patterns, they are also plastic and can change. They can be reprocessed, recontextualized and transformed to create new patterns or schemas (Edelman, 1987, 1989; Modell, 1996, 2006; Wagner et al., 2004; Kandel, 2006; Mancia, 2006).

These presymbolic experiences can be accessed through dreamwork among other methods (Mancia, 2006). Dreams can symbolically transform these preverbal, unconscious experiences into images so we may gain access, even without direct recollection. Mancia cites dream researcher Robert Stickgold et al. (2000) for support that implicit memories can be stored and then appear in dreams. The work of EI helps the patient make deep contact with these presymbolic memories by experiencing the dream images in her body.

The relationship between these early autobiographical memories and the imagination is explored by Modell (2006). We can experience these early memories with greater or lesser degrees of imagination; we can view the present with open curiosity and the ability to see novel meaning while still seeing links to the past or experience the present as merely a repeat of the past, leading to rigid enactment of dysfunctional, repetitive patterns.

Memory is linked to category formation (Edelman, 1989; Modell, 2006). Modell argues that our early, unconscious autobiographical memories form potential categories, and these categories are linked to consciousness by metaphor (Lakoff & Johnson, 1999).[3] Metaphor, because it is a form of cognition, can interpret unconscious memory. If our metaphors are fluid, we can view the present with openness and flexibility. Modell writes, "Metaphor not only *transfers* meaning between different domains, but (also) by means of novel re-combinations, metaphor can also *transform* meaning and generate new perceptions. Imagination could not exist without this re-combinatory metaphoric process" (2006, p. 27). Very much in line with EI, Modell refers to a "corporeal imagination," for example, expressed in the up/down dichotomy of "our spirits are up" and "he had a down day." George Lakoff (1993) suggests these metaphors come from bodily experiences. When we are drooping, we feel sad, but when we stand tall, we usually feel good.

Trauma and chronic stress can break down the metaphoric process, creating a foreclosed or frozen metaphoric process; the present becomes equated with the past. Modell (1996) therefore concludes that the compulsion to repeat is a function of memory, a rigid linking of the present with the past, and not the death instinct, as Freud (1920) postulated. Hence, as Mitchell (1993, p. 222) states, "psychopathology might well be considered a failure of imagination," the inability to create and/or experience the present in novel ways not predetermined by old, dysfunctional patterns.

This view of memory as a process of continual recategorization and not as a store of fixed attributes (Edelman, 1987) is similar to ideas developed by Freud that were later ignored. Freud (1895, 1909; Masson, 1985) stated that the failure of *Nachträeglichkeit*, defined by Modell (1996) as the ability to retranscribe or recontextualize memory in light of advancing developmental stages and subsequent experience, is the basis of psychopathology. As EI helps the patient transition from a foreclosed to a more open use of metaphor, it facilitates *Nachträeglichkeit*, allowing memory to be recontextualized and transformed.

Transformation and the alchemical therapist

Influenced by James Hillman who uses alchemical metaphors to describe the psychotherapeutic process, Bosnak's dream technique is based on metaphors derived from alchemy. In addition to being an early forerunner of modern chemistry, alchemy is a philosophical system of spiritual transformation, involving the expansion of consciousness and the development of insight and intuition through images. Although alchemy has been discredited for years, it is now viewed, in a metaphorical sense, as a path to help mankind return to the nonphysical world from a preoccupation with the physical. Historians are becoming aware of the connection between alchemy and the evolution of science and philosophy as well to mystical movements, such as Kabbala and spiritualism. Hillman views the poetic, metaphorical language of alchemy as itself therapeutic.

Working primarily in the Middle Ages and Renaissance, alchemists attempted to turn base metals into gold. However, just as Bosnak views dream images as quasi-physical substances, the alchemist also worked with the quasi-physical, that is, with the *spirit* of the metals.[4] Metals were seen as "bodies," alive with spirit and soul. According to the alchemists, each metal wants to return to its highest state (silver or gold), much like a patient's wish to actualize. Focusing on the release of the *spirit* of the metal rather than the concrete metal itself, the alchemist worked to reveal the metal's alien intelligence as he interacted with the metal. The dreamworker and dreamer attempt the same. All images in the dream are thought to be alive, not just a frightened person or a lively cat but also the waves in the ocean, a light bulb, the driving rain. As the dreamer works the images, he expands his imagination and enters a higher state.

In alchemy, degrees of physical and psychological transformation are represented by color. Hillman (2009) applies this to the psychotherapeutic process; the same understanding can be applied to EI. The successful psychological journey begins with *green*, the state of innocence when the patient is not even aware of a problem and then moves to *black* or darkness and chaos. Analogous versions are found in the biblical and Kabbalistic myths of creation, in which an original state of bliss or purity is shattered and man must venture into the unknown, into the darkness. It is here the process of change begins. Without the pessimism and helplessness of the black, the alchemical process cannot proceed.

Next comes the *white or silver*, which facilitates reflection and the ability to take on multiple perspectives. This awareness interrupts the compulsions of the black, much as mindful reflection can, at times, help a patient emerge from depression. Then there is a *yellowing* or a thickening, as the *white* image is put into the earth to ferment, equivalent to the "working through" process in therapy. The patient solidifies his gains.

Finally, the patient reaches the *red*. He or she can now move out into the world seeing subtleties of light and dark while retaining a sense of faith and optimism. This describes the alchemical transformation, the "healing" of the metal as well as the successful journey of the patient. This is a cyclical process. As new challenges are met, the journey is repeated.

Likewise, the dreamer has to pass through these stages. As the dreamer embodies habitual and alien images, he experiences a mixture of *green* and *black*, of naiveté and darkness. Then through the creation and practice of the composite, new intelligences emerge. Practicing the composite helps the dreamer consciously and unconsciously move to higher stages of reflection (*white*) and working through (*yellow*) and finally, create new networks as he reaches the *red*: vitality, passion and creativity. This may happen slowly, over the course of long periods of dreamwork and if the work continues, will be repeated again and again.

Technique of embodied imagination, or "knowing" by imagination

I now turn to a detailed discussion of the clinical technique itself.[5] To begin, the therapist encourages the patient to enter a waking hypnagogic state, a state naturally experienced while falling asleep, by having the patient close her or his eyes and engage in a brief relaxation technique[6] and then a body scan.[7,8] The therapist also enters the hypnagogic or reverie state and does the same exercise. Both participants hold, what Bosnak (2008) terms, a simultaneous dual consciousness, that is, they are completely immersed in the various images in the dream yet are also aware of themselves as separate. The therapist holds this simultaneous dual consciousness even more completely because she or he must plan a strategy for working the dream and guiding the patient while keeping track of time. To reiterate, the dream that is worked does not emerge from the hypnagogic state but is a remembered dream that the patient brings to the session.

The patient tells the remembered dream to the therapist in the present tense, as if it is happening right then. The therapist listens carefully. The patient does not read the dream; she simply tells it. The therapist listens and does not take notes. The patient then associates to the dream and retells it.

During the first telling, the therapist notices the feelings in his own body, as evoked by the patient's dream. When the patient tells her dream for the second time, the therapist forms a strategy and decides which images to work and in what order. Usually there are several strong images in a dream. The therapist typically chooses one that represents the "habitual self," possibly another "safe" image if the habitual image is not safe, and then one or two others, so-called alien intelligences, which are strong and contradictory to the habitual self. Although the therapist usually chooses the images, he can also do this in collaboration with the patient. However, this risks pulling the patient out of the hypnagogic state, whereas the therapist is more aware of his dual consciousness. Regardless, if the patient feels an important image is being left out, she should feel free to tell the therapist so the image can be included.

The therapist then guides the patient to slowly embody various images in the dream, that is, to "enter" the image, and use her imagination to feel it in her body. For example, a patient might describe a woman in an image as "standing, looking very tired." The therapist inquires, "Is she erect or slouching?" "Where in her body does she feel that slouch? OK, in the shoulders. Now can *you* try and sense into that slouch?" and so on. This helps the patient connect with the bodily feelings in the selected images. Working at the bodily level is paramount, as we want to be as immersed as much as possible in the unconscious, which is housed in the body and its habits.

The patient is guided to group these selected images together into a "composite," which is a combination of the key images. She practices reexperiencing them in session: feeling them in her body, imagining them backward and forward. After the session the patient practices the composite for 20 minutes daily, the length of time recommended by Kosslyn and Moulton (2009) as optimal for mental practice that will affect behavior. This can be broken up into several minutes a number of times a day. At first the patient imagines the images in a series but eventually tries to imagine them almost simultaneously. This continues for several weeks after the session.

Habitual patterns are very strong and will reassert themselves unless countered with concerted effort. Practicing the composite holds it in memory and helps stabilize the new emotional learning. Hebb's phrase – neurons that fire together wire together – applies (Hebb, 1949). A synapse strengthens when the neurons it connects repeatedly fire together. This creates patterns of neural activity through which genuine "thirds" emerge, that is, functional entities not reducible to the sum of their parts (Kaag, 2009). As the reader is aware, the "third" Kaag discusses in terms of the creation of new neuronal structures parallels the "third" discussed in psychoanalysis.

It is also very important to choose images that evoke emotion so as to activate the hormonal system of emotionally enhanced memory encoding. Emotional arousal releases adrenal stress hormones that enhance the memory of the experience (McGaugh & Roozendaal, 2002; Cahill & Alkire, 2003). Events that evoke emotional responses are likely to be important for survival and so are more important to remember, which the hormonal mechanism promotes.

Embodied imagination resolves creative insecurities

When faced with insecurity and uncertainty, as I was when writing Chapter 5 on biology, which is not my area of expertise, I turn to a technique of EI called "incubation," an approach frequently used to foster creative projects. When I initially approached Chapter 5, I had many doubts. Maybe a medical person should write this? Maybe I don't fully understand the concepts? Maybe I will be laughed at for pretending to be something I'm not? However, and this is very important, I also felt excitement about exploring new territory and potentially seeing psychotherapy from a new perspective.

My fellow LA3 dream worker, Swedish director and playwright Pelle Nordin, guided me in the incubation process, which takes a memory related to the creative project and works it as a dream. The participant embodies the images in the memory and forms a composite (a collection of two to four embodied images chosen from the memory). Then he or she practices the composite for several weeks after the session. This stimulates subsequent dreams that address the problem.

To begin this process of incubation, I tried to think about Chapter 5 as a living entity, akin to a character in a play. Actors use this type of incubation to gain insight into their character.[9] I combined memories about a recent medical scare with a mentor's criticism of the ideas for the chapter to create an incubation. I used the incubation composite both to spark subsequent dreams as well as to inspire me each time I began writing.

To give more in the way of explanation, concerning the medical scare, I had gotten a CT scan required for a minor surgical procedure. There was an incidental finding on the scan that required me to get an MRI and see a surgeon, who told me I needed a major operation. I was quite frightened by this. I then consulted one of the chief medical experts in the field for a second opinion. He explained, including showing me the MRI images in great detail, how my body was taking care of it *on its own* and that I definitely didn't need an operation (straight out of Chapter 5, which discusses biological imagination and how the body frequently repairs itself!). The memory of this relief – the moment I tell my husband I no longer need an operation – is the first anchor point of the composite. Second, I remember a conversation with a former mentor who was very critical of some of my initial ideas for the chapter, and I embody him. This is the second point of the composite. Third, I embody the chapter itself as a young horse, buried under a huge mound of hay, terrified, struggling to stand up and find some air to breathe. (I have bolded the embodied aspect of each image.)

My composite:

(1) **I feel awe and energy in the air in my lungs, going up the back of my head into my eyes** as I talk to my husband on the phone and tell him I don't need an operation. I explain how I saw the MRI images. I have seen the secret, seen inside my body. It's a revelation. Like winning the lottery. The next 6 months are mine – no operation!

(2) **A call to battle. I feel this going up the spine of my former mentor who is critical of the chapter. He holds his head high and looks at me in a challenging manner.** For him, this is war! The chapter is a stupid idea and has to be stopped.

(3) **The terror of the horse, twisting and turning his head, has to get air, get up and out from under the hay. He has to live!**

Working this composite – that is practicing it and feeling it in the body – relaxed me and helped waylay doubt. I could focus more clearly and let Chapter 5 breathe and speak for itself. I also refound my own voice and could see above the data I had accumulated to focus on clarifying patterns regarding subsets of the imagination, which I added to Chapter 1. The delineation of the various types of imagination helped provide a connecting, unifying thread for the book. I had many dreams following the incubation, some of which I worked using EI, which continued to help me with the writing.

Clinical use of embodied imagination

As I integrate EI into my practice, I find varied responses among patients. Some are very enthusiastic and feel excited to be collaborating on a unique method of working so directly with the unconscious. Others are more neutral but willing to give it a try. These patients seem to particularly enjoy that we both enter the hypnagogic state. This creates a feeling of working very closely together.

Another group, however, is more negative and after trying it once, choose not to pursue this way of working. Although my sample is very small, it appears that, in some cases, patients who actively reject this approach are more self-conscious about their bodies and sexuality and/or frightened of the unexpected eruption of aggression. This technique may not be appropriate for these patients, or at least not until they are more comfortable.[10] Other patients simply prefer more traditional methods of dreamwork.

Also, there is the issue of how much to talk about "meaning." EI tends to favor the patient practicing the composite and letting it "cook," that is, have change take place unconsciously in the body, without discussing meaning. It can be argued that bringing the process to consciousness interferes with this unconscious change. However, this approach is counterintuitive for most therapists. A good balance might be to have the patient practice the composite for a week or two and then discuss meaning, if this approach works for the treatment. At times, the patient herself may introduce interpretative material, especially in the discussion right after the dream is worked. Again, if the dreamworker feels it is very important to keep the work on the implicit level only, she can say so and indicate they can speak about meaning several weeks later, after the practice work on the composite is completed. Other times, the dreamworker may find it helpful to incorporate the interpretative work right then.

As mentioned, Bosnak (2008) uses alchemical terms and concepts in a metaphorical and allegorical sense to describe his EI work. The concept of "cooking the composite" is taken from this. He describes alchemy as "a peculiar mixture of chemistry and the imagination" (2008, p. 74). The alchemists saw the metals they worked with as having soul and possessing intelligence. Using fire, they processed ("cooked") the metals to reveal this intelligence and create a transformation. In EI, as he practices the composite, the patient "cooks" or "processes" his dream images to create change.

Clinical examples

The following dream is from a patient, Ms. D, a 35-year-old woman who is a gifted singer and sculptor. Ms. D and I have been working together for several years, and she continues to struggle with fully expressing her creativity.

Her father, a volatile, creative man, was also a singer, but for various reasons, his creativity was stifled. The following is an example of a dream that was brought up midway in the session and could only be worked for 25 minutes. Although this is a short period of time for this effort, I felt we were able to cover the main images and put them together as a composite. For the reader's convenience, I am bolding the images that will be used in the composite.

Dream: *Ms. D sees a* ***healthy baby*** *crawling into a hole in the wall, about to go in and disappear. She goes over to it and,* ***with her strong arms, stops it****. Then, she is in her mother's house, and it is very old and dusty looking, cluttered with collectibles all over. She hears a* ***toy piano*** *playing, and it seems to be playing by itself. Then when she walks closer, the keys are being depressed but there is no sound. Maybe a ghost is playing it. She is beginning to get scared. Then she sees a young child who appears "neutral" but looks like a child on a Twilight Zone episode that can change adults and cause harm if they do something he doesn't like. Then she turns, and a door to the cabinet that held her father's old 45s and 78s opens by itself.* ***Then the front door opens,*** *and she is getting more and more terrified.* ***She tries to scream but can't and just shakes her head as if she is getting demented****.*

Ms. D's association to the toy piano was that she has been neglecting her singing voice and feels creatively blocked. She also identified the toy piano as representing her father's inability to continue with his singing, something that had always upset the patient. She discussed her bond with her father – he was a creative force – but also her fear of his volatility despite his being loving toward her.

From embodying the images in the dream, the following composite developed: (1) the normal, active baby that with its **whole healthy body is crawling to a goal, unafraid**. The baby feels this in **his entire body;** (2) Ms. D's **strong arms stopping the baby from getting hurt;** (3) the **dusty old toy piano** that has been neglected and is playing a plaintive sound before it loses its voice. This is felt in the **toy piano, in its silence**; and (4) **the frightening front door**. This is experienced in **her silent scream and her shaking head.** Then we practiced this composite, feeling and repeating the images backward and forward, until they were experienced almost simultaneously. In the composite, the health of the baby and Ms. D's strong, sturdy arms modulate her terror, anger and sadness that her creativity has been suppressed.

From an interpretative or meaning perspective, this dream suggests the patient's wish to "sing" as well as her intense fear/anxiety (she is extremely frightened as the front door opens). She has considerable strength (healthy baby, strong capable arms) but feels both she and her father have been stifled (the dusty toy piano that cannot make sounds). She also wants the power to retaliate for being stifled (child who can cause harm). In this instance, I did not discuss the possible meanings of the dream but just had the patient practice the composite, and this was successful. In other instances, it might be appropriate to do interpretative work after the composite has been practiced.

In subsequent sessions, Ms. D discussed the dream and how she continued to use the images and work the composite. After this dream, she had several other dreams concerning fears of retaliation from her family for expressing her creativity. These were all worked in many sessions, again following this technique. She addressed her neglect of her voice and began singing lessons again. Using her father's Greek heritage as the basis for projects, she developed several new ideas for vocal performing. The dreamwork also facilitated her work as a sculptor. She is moving forward in producing her art and arranging venues for exhibitions.

The next example further illustrates how this technique can help with anxiety. Although extremely competent, 50-year-old Ms. C has considerable anxiety about job performance. She has been in therapy for several years. At the time of this dream, she was especially anxious about a yearly event she organizes, although managing this event has always created anxiety for her. This year, company politics surrounding the event were making it especially difficult.

She told this dream about a week before the event.

Dream: *Ms. C was with a group of people in her office. They were supposed to remain in her office to do their work in a contained, intense setting. Yet they were thinking of continuing it outside the office.* ***One of the men in the group*** *said in a firm, calm, direct manner, "No, that isn't right. We shouldn't do this." He has* ***a military bearing****. Then Ms. C was outside with Susan, another member of the group.* ***Susan was very anxious****. Her arms were flailing around. It was cold and rainy. Susan said she was working for the mayor and had to be at the St. Patrick's Day Parade. Susan was almost in a panic as she was saying this, as if a great deal was at stake. She could lose her job if something went wrong. Then the scene changed and Ms. C and Susan were back in the office.* ***Susan was sitting at a piano, playing and beginning to calm down****.*

As we worked the dream, the following composite emerged: (1) the man who is confident, firm, military-like and he feels this in his back and his spine; (2) Susan who is panicked and feels this in her pounding heart; and (3) Susan who is in the flow of practicing and has focus, feeling this in her mind and the movement of her arms. We practiced this composite in session until Ms. C felt confident that she could do it on her own.

I sensed that if Ms. C practiced this and felt these images in her body, it would help calm her. This composite gave her access to her anxiety as well as several ways to modulate it. Ms. C did practice this composite, and for the first time since she has been organizing and leading this complex annual event, she was not overwhelmed with anxiety about its preparation and execution. She said she was mostly calm throughout the planning and during the event itself, and she attributed this, in part, to the dreamwork.

I have used this technique for many other clinical issues, including problems with depression, separation anxiety and fears concerning sexuality. It has also helped increase mindfulness regarding weight issues. This is not to suggest that the technique is limited to these issues, but just that this is my clinical experience to date.

Personal experience with Embodied Imagination

In my EI training I regularly worked my dreams with a guide, either with a faculty member or with a colleague in the program. EI can be incorporated into ongoing psychotherapeutic treatment or used as a "stand alone" practice. The dreams I discuss below are in the latter context. I am "the dreamer," in the sense that I worked my dreams with a guide or "dream worker," but not in the context of ongoing therapy. The images were chosen by the guide, not by me.

Although participation in EI program is training and not psychotherapy, I have found the endeavor therapeutic. At the point I joined the program, I wanted to allow myself more leisure time to write, including poetry, play writing and songwriting even though becoming more creative and playful seemed, to the overworked and intellectualized parts of myself, an impossible task. As a result of regularly working my dreams and the dreams of my colleagues, I have been able to move forward and write in these various forms.

The following are several dreams of mine that I felt were key in helping me progress. In the first dream, I illustrate how I attempt to "enter" each image, that is, feel it in my body. One of the leaders of the program was my guide in working this dream.

The dream of the Crayola-colored dreadlocks

I am in a resort with many people, and one of my colleagues, A, is there with his wife. We all seem to be together and are going to a restaurant. A is angry because his wife is late. The rest of us go to the restaurant but A doesn't come. I am shocked that ***he can break the frame of the group's expectation*** *and not come with us. A and his wife come later. The table we sit down at is a mess. Debris from the previous meal is all over, seems like it was an Italian meal. We go to a different table to start.*

Then suddenly there is a man, a friend of a friend, who wants me to go with him to the playroom in his apartment building to be with his wife who is there with their two children. (She is someone I don't know well, and I don't have a "sense" of her.) I go to the playroom with him, and she's there. She has a weird hairpiece. It ***is a ponytail of dreadlocks in different bright primary Crayola colors****. These are very bright and vivid in the context of a more mutely colored dream.*

Then this man has a problem, and he asks me to go get something for him. He stays in the playroom with his wife and children. I realize I didn't bring my keys, which I need. I had to go home to get them, and it's getting dark. ***I am tired. I think, "I do so much. No one knows all I do."***

In working the dream, the first image we focused on was that of my colleague, A, who broke the frame. I felt a mixture of envy and admiration that he was able to do this. As I entered this image, I was able to feel his independence, his ability to go his own way, and I felt this in my torso. The breaking of the frame is needed for creative work to begin.

Then I was guided to the dreadlocks. Powerful and playful at the same time, they say, "I am here!" It is fitting that they are on the body of someone I don't have a "sense" of, as this claim to be seen is a foreign idea to me. I try to enter this presence as well and laugh and giggle while I am in it. I feel her dreadlocks on her head. Commanding, a strong childlike presence. I feel captured by her electricity and childlike wonder.

I am also aware of the play on words. I dread giving up even a small amount of my clinical work to make time for creative work. At the same time, I feel "locked" into that way of being, the overwork, and I dread that as well. This arresting presence of the dreads is perhaps another ingredient of creativity – the "I am here," emphatic, confident, bold statement – brought to me in the body of someone I don't understand. Entering this presence was difficult for me, and it took continual practice.

Then the last image I worked was my tired habitual self who is weary and feels unappreciated. I feel this strongly in my neck and shoulders, as I walk along the slowly darkening street. I am so very tired and resigned.

I form a composite of these three images, trying to imagine them at the same time, including the bodily sensations. I replay this in my mind for the next few weeks. My habitually tired and exhausted self is potentially mingling with the charismatic and arresting presences to create a new formation.

The next night, I had the dream below, which I experienced as a hopeful and optimistic follow-up.

My hand goes through walls

I am trying to get out of my triple-locked hotel room. I had been afraid someone would come in so I had triple-locked it. I was also afraid the very heavy door would hit my fingers when I shut it. Now I can open the door by putting my hand through the wall very easily and moving it around to the handle. The concrete wall becomes a lighter color and the material almost translucent but yet not. It is still a kind of wall but I can easily put my hand through it.

The almost translucent material of the wall seems like the inside of a fruit, lifegiving. I am no longer bound by concrete. Yet it is still a wall. I still have boundaries but there is more fluidity and less blocking. When I triple-locked the door in the dream, I was afraid of intruders – rapists or thieves – so I "over-locked" it. Now I can open it easily. I have the feeling I can "do it." I can easily and effortlessly break through my multilocked door. It can happen. I can be more "free."

The dreams reported above began a period of about 10 weeks when my dreams revolved around these themes. During that time, I became increasingly focused and energetic and began work on a variety of writing projects. I felt less critical of myself, and that, if I put effort into it, I can accomplish entry into a more creative life. I embraced the idea of reducing my clinical schedule, even though before I was "dreading" any kind of change in that regard. To use Modell's terms, the dreamwork increased my ability for open rather than closed metaphor. I was able to see more broadly and boldly.

What changed? The weary exhaustion of the downtrodden habitual self was less in evidence and replaced with more vitality, confidence and increased creativity. Possibly the early unconscious "knowings"' of the victimized, self-sacrificing self had altered to form a more effective and spontaneous self.

During this period, I was motivated to seek help for a chronic neck problem that caused intense headaches. Now, actually and symbolically, I am largely pain free. This is not to say that all my anxieties are solved, but rather, this likely represents a period of work that has come to a successful close – only to be followed by a new series of dreams that will deepen this work and begin new work. I do, however, feel a physiological, emotional and behavioral change.

Dreaming and creativity

Many regard dreaming as the mental state most likely to foster creativity (Hobson, 1988). Stickgold et al. (2001) review brain activity during REM dreaming. We gain access to emotions without the cognitive controls normally present, networks of associated memories that we cannot normally access. In REM, the brain is looking for new ways to connect these associative networks, allowing us to form novel associations. Stickgold et al. hypothesize that the brain identifies and evaluates these new connections, which can lead either to a strengthening or weakening of associations. If a new association is strengthened sufficiently, it gets laid down as new memory. This is the neurological correlate of a new idea or possibility for the patient.

Experimental support is provided by Ullrich Wagner and colleagues (2004) who conclude that sleep, by restructuring memory representations, facilitates insight. They write that sleep "not only strengthens memory traces quantitatively, but can also 'catalyze' mental restructuring, thereby setting the stage for the emergence of insight" (Wagner et al., 2004, p. 354). Mark Blechner also explores this dream processing which he calls "oneiric Darwinism: to create 'thought mutations' – new ideas and objects, created through partially random processes – that the mind can then retain if useful or reject if useless" (Blechner, 2013, p. 260).

Regarding the emergence of insight, Paolo Mazzarello (2000) reviews several famous scientific insights reported as a result of dreaming. August Kekulé discovered the ring structure of benzene, an important organic chemical compound, with ideas developed from a dream image. The Nobel Prize winner Otto Loewi reported that he woke up from a dream with the essential idea for an experimental confirmation of his theory of chemical neurotransmission. Dmitri Mendeleyev, who laid out the periodic table of chemical elements, reported that he grasped the critical underlying rule from a dream, after many unsuccessful attempts while awake.

As an explanation, Mazzarello cites the discoveries of Pierre Maquet and colleagues (2000) that memory traces from waking life are processed during REM sleep. From these findings Mazzarello (2000) suggests that a new concept, perhaps only hinted at when awake, can sometimes be better conveyed in a dream when the memory traces are reactivated and processed. The new idea then comes to consciousness as a remembered dream. Maquet and colleagues suggest that REM sleep may be a privileged period for learning, not just in the child's brain but in the adult's as well. New memories can be tenuous and easily disrupted by the learning of other information, preventing long-term memory consolidation. In REM there is a neuromodular shift to a high level of the neurotransmitter acetylcholine. This elevated level of cholinergic activity is probably necessary for brain plasticity and may help consolidate new learning (Maquet et al., 2000).[11]

There are several different possible processes at work. One is that as a result of sleep and dreaming, we can awaken with an "aha" experience where we suddenly find the key to a particular problem embedded in the dream we remember. It may come to us fully formed "Oh that's how I have to approach it!" or as an image that is easily understood, as in the example in Chapter 4 of my dream image of the mermaid with the head of Joan Crawford.

On the other hand, dreams can have a number of images, some of which are unusual or bizarre and not immediately understandable, and the patient needs focused dreamwork before she can use them. In the work of EI, these unusual, novel images can be juxtaposed with images of the habitual self. This allows us access to the variety of ingredients needed to create new networks and bring these to consciousness.

To conclude, as therapists, we are called to expand the capacity for imagination in our patients and in ourselves. Bromberg writes, the therapeutic relationship can be thought of as "a journey in which two people must each loosen the rigidity of their dissociative 'truths' about self and other to allow 'imagination' to find its shared place" (Bromberg, 2013, p. 1). Our exploration of EI not only gives us a significant tool for expanding imagination but also greater insight into what is effective in creating therapeutic change.

As the chemist Kekulé said, talking with scientists about his discovery in 1865 of the structure of the benzene ring from a dream, "Let us learn to dream, gentlemen" (quoted in Modell, 2006, p. 28).

Notes

1 An earlier version of this chapter appeared in Domash (2016) and is gratefully reprinted with permission from Taylor & Francis.
2 Modell (2006, p. 27) defines metaphor as "a mapping or transfer of meaning between dissimilar domains (from a source domain to a target domain)," acknowledging the play of similarity and difference.
3 George Lakoff and Mark Johnson view metaphor as a form of cognition, part of the conceptual system underlying English. These conceptual metaphors are so interwoven into our language that we are usually not aware of them. Lakoff (1993, p. 78) gives the example of "Love is a journey." Many possible "spin-off" metaphors are possible. For example, "We've hit a dead-end" suggests trouble while "Look how far we've come" is more promising.
4 The information that follows on alchemy is based on lectures given by Robert Bosnak, LA3 Embodied Imagination, Malinalco MX, January 29, 2016 to February 1, 2016.
5 For a thorough discussion of the technique, see Bosnak (1996, 1998, 2008).
6 The relaxation technique might involve the therapist counting down from ten to one. With each recited number, the patient feels himself descending, as if in an elevator. This helps the patient reduce the "thinking" function, such as self-monitoring and self-censorship, and enter a more relaxed state.
7 The patient, using his imagination, scans his body for feelings from head to toe. The body scan gives the patient a sense of a baseline, as later the patient will be asked to "enter" the images and say where he experiences them in his body. It is important to note where he has sensations in his body before the work begins.
8 The purpose of the relaxation technique and body scan is for the patient to feel simultaneously relaxed and alert. Each practitioner is encouraged to develop her own style, as long as the patient has sufficient time to enter the hypnagogic state.
9 See Sonenberg, J. (2003). *Dreamwork for actors.* New York: Routledge.
10 It is also possible that these patients could use a modified approach, as Bromberg (2003) describes. Bromberg uses EI in his ongoing analytic work, although not with every patient. He does not use a "hard-nosed" (Bromberg, 2003, p. 701) hypnotic induction, which I infer to mean he does not use a formal relaxation technique or body scan so as not to interrupt the flow of the analytic work. Another modification might be to only work with an image of habitual consciousness, to help a patient acclimate to the technique.
11 The neurotransmitter acetylcholine has been recognized by memory researchers as a local enhancer of plasticity and as a consolidator of long-term memory (Power, 2004).

References

Blechner, M. (2013). New ways of conceptualizing and working with dreams. *Contemporary Psychoanalysis*, 49:259–275.

Bosnak, R. (1996). *Tracks in the wilderness of dreaming: Exploring interior landscape through practical dreamwork*. New York: Delacorte Press.

Bosnak, R. (1998). *A little course in dreams*. Boston, MA: Shambhala Press.

Bosnak, R. (2008). *Embodiment: Creative imagination in medicine, art and travel*. New York: Routledge.

Bromberg, P.M. (2003). On being one's own dream: Some reflections on Robert Bosnak's "Embodied Imagination." *Contemporary Psychoanalysis*, 39:697–710.

Bromberg, P.M. (2013). Hidden in plain sight: Thoughts on imagination and the lived unconscious. *Psychoanalytic Dialogues*, 23:1–14.

Cahill, L. & Alkire, M. (2003). Epinephrine enhancement of human memory consolidation: Interaction with arousal at encoding. *Neurobiology of Learning and Memory*, 79:194–198.

Cozolino, L. (2002). *The neuroscience of psychotherapy: Building and rebuilding the human brain*. New York: Norton.

Cozolino, L. (2006). *The neuroscience of human relationships: Attachment and the developing brain*. New York: Norton.

Darwin, C. (1879/2004). *The descent of man*. New York: Penguin.

Domash, L. (2016). Dreamwork and transformation: Facilitating therapeutic change using embodied imagination. *Contemporary Psychoanalysis*, 52(3):1–24.

Edelman, G. (1987). *Neural Darwinism*. New York: Basic Books.

Edelman, G. (1989). *The remembered present: A biological theory of consciousness*. New York: Basic Books.

Freud, S. (1895). Project for a scientific psychology. *Standard Edition*, 1:281–391.

Freud, S. (1909). Notes upon a case of obsessional neurosis. *Standard Edition*, 10:153–249.

Freud, S. (1920). Beyond the pleasure principle. *Standard Edition*, 1:1–64.

Ginot, E. (2007). Intersubjectivity and neuroscience: Understanding enactments and their therapeutic significance within emerging paradigms. *Psychoanalytic Psychology*, 24:317–332.

Ginot, E. (2015). *The neuropsychology of the unconscious: Integrating brain and mind in psychotherapy*. New York: Norton.

Hebb, D. (1949). *The organization of behavior: A neuropsychological theory*. New York: John Wiley.

Hillman, J. (2009). *Alchemical psychology: Uniform edition of the writings of James Hillman, Vol. 5*. Thompson, CT: Spring Publications.

Hobson, J.A. (1988). *The dreaming brain*. New York: Basic Books.

Kaag, J. (2009). The neurological dynamics of the imagination. *Phenomenology and Cognitive Sciences*, 8:183–204.

Kandel, E.R. (2006). *In search of memory: The emergence of a new science of mind*. New York: Norton.

Kosslyn, S. & Moulton, S. (2009). Mental imagery and implicit memory. In K.D. Markman, W.M.P. Klein & J.A. Suhr (Eds.), *Handbook of imagination and mental stimulation* (pp. 35–51). New York: Psychology Press.

Lakoff, G. (1993). How metaphor structures dreams: The theory of conceptual metaphor applied to dream analysis. *Dreaming*, 3:77–98.

Lakoff, G. & Johnson, M. (1999). *Philosophy in the flesh*. New York: Basic Books.

Mancia, M. (2006). Implicit memory and early unrepressed unconscious: Their role in the therapeutic process (How the neurosciences can contribute to psychoanalysis). *International Journal of Psychoanalysis*, 87:83–103.

Maquet, P., Laureys, S., Peigneux, P., Fuchs, S., Petiau, C., Phillips, C., Aerts, J., Del Fiore, G., Degueldre, C., Meulemans, T., Luxen, A., Franck, G., Van der Linden, M., Smith, C. & Cleeremans, A. (2000). Experience-dependent changes in cerebral activation during REM sleep. *Nature Neuroscience*, 3(8):831–836.

Masson, J.M. (1985). *The complete letters of Sigmund Freud to Wilhelm Fliess*. Cambridge, MA: Harvard University Press.

Mazzarello, P. (2000). What dreams may come? *Nature*, 408:523.

McGaugh, J. & Roozendaal, B. (2002). Role of adrenal stress hormones in forming lasting memories in the brain. *Current Opinion in Neurobiology*, 12:205–210.

Mitchell, S. (1993). *Hope and dread in psychoanalysis*. New York: Basic Books.

Modell, A. (1996). *Other times, other realities: Toward a theory of psychoanalytic treatment*. Cambridge, MA: Harvard University Press.

Modell, A. (2006). *Imagination and the meaningful brain*. Cambridge, MA: MIT Press.

Modell, A. (April 13, 2008). The unconscious as a knowledge processing center. 28th Annual Spring Meeting of the Division of Psychoanalysis (39) of the American Psychological Association, *Knowing, Not Knowing and Sort-of-Knowing: Psychoanalysis and the Experience of Uncertainty*, New York City, NY.

Modell, A. (2009). Metaphor – The bridge between feelings and knowledge. *Psychological Inquiry*, 29:6–11.

Power, A.E. (2004). Slow-wave sleep, acetylcholine, and memory consolidation. *Proceedings of the National academy of Sciences USA*, 101(7):1795–1796.

Schore, A.N. (1994). *Affect regulation and the origins of the self: The neurology of emotional development*. Hillsdale, NJ: Erlbaum.

Schore, A.N. (2005). A neuropsychoanalytic viewpoint: Commentary on paper by Steven H. Knoblauch. *Psychoanalytic Dialogues*, 15:829–854.

Siegel, D. (1999). *The developing mind: How relationships and the brain interact to shape who we are*. New York: Guilford.

Siegel, D. (2007). *The mindful brain*. New York: Norton.

Stickgold, R., Malia, A., Maguire, D., Roddenberry, D. & O'Connor, M. (2000). Replaying the game: Hypnagogic images in normals and amnesics. *Science*, 290(5490):350–353.

Stickgold, R., Hobson, J.A., Fosse, R. & Fosse, M. (2001). Sleep, learning, and dreams: Off-line memory reprocessing. *Science*, 294(5544):1052–1057.

Taussig, M. (1993). *Mimesis and alterity: A particular history of the senses*. New York: Routledge.

Wagner, U., Gais, S., Haider, H., Verieger, R. & Born, J. (2004). Sleep inspires insight. *Nature*, 427:352–355.

Chapter 7

Trauma

Imagination interrupted[1]

Embodied imagination and trauma

Dreams are a potentially creative space for traumatized patients. When successful, one of the functions of dreaming is to contextualize trauma and weave it into the psychological system as a whole (Hartmann, 2001). Psychiatrist and dream researcher Ernest Hartmann bases his conclusions on the study of thousands of posttraumatic dreams. Those individuals who develop PTSD from trauma tend to represent the trauma in dreams in fixed repetitive ways, while those who do not develop PTSD gradually alter aspects of the traumatic event in their dreams, introducing other material from their life. The latter becomes possible because dreams can, in many cases, allow broader emotional connections to be made than when awake, allowing the trauma to become metabolized (Hartmann, 2001).

Inspired by Hartmann's underlying premise that imagination/dreaming can help process trauma, Bosnak devised dream methods to work with trauma. He began to focus on features of the dream that are different from how the dreamer remembers the actual event. This approach creates space for imaginative representations, similar to individuals who introduced new elements into their dreams and did not develop PTSD. As the patient introduces new material and views the trauma from different perspectives, she develops flexibility and gains strength to stop the repetitive reliving of the trauma. It no longer remains heavy in the body and mind, undigested.

From this, Bosnak developed a system of artificial flashbacks or memories to work with trauma. In the context of a safe relationship with the therapist, the patient chooses a memory of a traumatic event. In a state of dual consciousness, she is led into the memory (and therefore the trauma) but also knows she has created the flashback, and it is only a memory. The flashback is then worked as a dream, again with an emphasis on any new details that are different from how the person remembers the actual event. Working with a memory is especially helpful as memories may be more accessible to patients than dreams, which can be evanescent. This initial memory work will frequently spark a series of dreams that help the patient continue to metabolize the trauma.

An additional technique is to find a safe image in the dream and view the trauma from the point of view of the safe image, which reduces the possibility of retraumatization. For example, if it is a rape scene, the patient can view and embody this not from the point of view of the person being raped but from a safe object in the room, such as a lamp in the dream giving off soft light. (In EI inanimate objects are seen as having presence and perspective just as much as animate beings.) Viewing the trauma from the perspective of a safe image lessens the impact and makes it more tolerable.

The following is an account of a very ill man hospitalized with advanced rectal cancer, whom Bosnak (2008) names the Cat Dreamer. This patient had completely withdrawn and would not cooperate with treatment or communicate, even with his wife. All sense of wanting or agency was lost. However, in this dream, he introduces a new safe image into his experience:

> I am in a strange room in a city. I'm lying on a couch. In the back of the room, behind the TV I see two lights. At first I think it is the traffic outside. But then I realize it is a cat. I see the cat move around the room. I call for my wife, but she isn't there. This is strange because my wife is usually around. Then I call for my son. He is not there either. I am alone in the room with the cat.
>
> (Bosnak, 2008, p. 51)

The patient has inserted a new element, the cat, into his trauma. Neither his wife, who is usually with him, nor his son, is in the room – only the cat. He loves cats and has one at home, although he has never seen this cat before.

At first when the patient begins to explore the dream, he feels stiff and flat. Then he gradually observes how gracefully the cat moves. Bosnak encourages the patient to feel into his body and mimic the movements of the cat. The more the patient's body state becomes like the cat, the more he feels the cat's energy. Bosnak works with the patient over a series of sessions, as the energy of the cat continues to infuse him. After this dreamwork, the patient's spirits improve. He becomes more communicative and cooperates with treatment. He has a much better quality of life until, sadly, his death later in the year. In this example, through the process of mimesis, the Cat Dreamer was able to imitate and identify with the cat and thereby introduce a new, vital aspect of experience into his consciousness.

Another related example of working with trauma is a dream from writer and shaman Narandja Eagelson, an esteemed colleague from our LA3 Embodied Imagination Group. I led the group work on this particular dream. Narandja's dream has a traumatic element and three relatively "safe" images. The traumatic element involves repetitive fears from her childhood in poverty-stricken rural Croatia where food was scare. As a young child, she was burdened by many responsibilities on her family's small farm and would worry she might do the wrong thing and incur the anger of the adults who were depending on her. Her family's lineage in the Balkan peninsula dates back 10,000 years, and they have lived in what is now Croatia for at least 600. These fears about working the land and caring for the animals have been passed down for countless generations.

After listening to the below dream, my goal was to reduce Narandja's feeling of panic and fear, which becomes evident at the end of the dream. I have bolded the images in the dream that will be used in the composite to make it clearer for the reader.

Dream: I am traveling away from my home with my sister and Gary. It is nightfall. Feel sadness and grief because we have not found what we are looking for but it is time to rest. I follow Gary and my sister under a Roman arch into a monastery or castle. Here I start to feel ***a shield in my chest, which is mirrored in a shield in the castle. These shields are like capsules that hold my chest together and give me relief from the sadness and grief****. I will sleep and rest.* ***I am free for the night****.*

I walk up the wide stone stairs and hear monastic chanting music from below. The ***music is certain of its repeating pattern and is not influenced by others. It has certainty****. You can feel the music in the round disc billowing up from below.*

Then I walk right and see the room where there are narrow beds to sleep. I see my two dogs running past the other way. I call to them. As I lay down on the bed, they come in. One of them, Kashi, lies down on my stomach with his head on my chest. He relaxes and I feel how quickly he is drifting into wonderful sleep. ***A soft cloud of forgetting. A letting go in his sinew, muscles, bones. His eyes are full of trust.***

Then I start to think: Did I feed the dogs? Who is feeding them? I can't remember. They have to be fed. Am I worthy of Kashi's trust? Have I done my job? ***Did I betray him?*** *This would be unforgivable. They are like babies. Innocents.* ***I feel panic. An acid burning – a choking in my ears, throat and chest.***

The composite is:

1 the shield in the chest mirrored in the shield in the castle. Relief from sadness and grief. Free for the night.
2 the certainty in the repeating pattern of the music. Not affected by others.
3 letting go in the sinews, muscles, bones and eyes. Soft cloud of forgetting.
4 acid burning panic in the ears, throat and chest. Did I break the trust? Am I worthy?

The trauma is represented in the last image by the acid burning panic in the dreamer's body. Has she fed her dogs? She can't remember. Has she betrayed Kashi's trust? Animals and children cannot be neglected. They must be fed! Narandja became very upset and emotional during this fourth anchor.

After working the dream, the dreamworker frequently asks the dreamer if any new image has come up, any emergent phenomenon. Narandja reported an image of a bolt of lightning, which would destroy everything. In the ensuing discussion, Narandja herself introduced some interpretative work. She thought the fourth anchor represented repetitive fears from her childhood in rural Croatia where food was scare. Among many responsibilities, her job was to care for and feed the animals, on which the family depended for food.

She said that still, panic around these feelings can completely take over like a bolt of lightning that will destroy everything. However, she herself has introduced **three new images** into the dream environment: the feeling of protection in the shields, the certainty of the music billowing up (not being influenced by others) and Kashi's letting go into relaxed sleep. None of these – a sense of protection, certainty or relaxation – had been present at the time of the original trauma. As she practices the composite, Narandja will work to strengthen the first three images. These images can recontextualize, reframe and modulate the panic at the end, just as the lively cat modified the flat, stiff image of the Cat Dreamer. Essentially in this work, we are helping the dreamer do what Hartmann observed in the subjects who were able on their own to recontextualize or metabolize their trauma. By working the dream and practicing the composite, Narandja is taking a congealed or fixed trauma (the fourth anchor) and modifying/changing it by combining it with newly introduced safe images. As she practices the composite, Narandja will push the system to the edge of chaos and a qualitatively new reality may be created.

Ogden (2010) discusses several types of thinking, among which are dream thinking and transformative thinking, both of which generate psychological growth. (When Ogden discusses thinking, he is always referring to thinking *and* feeling.) Dream thinking views emotional experience from multiple vantage points at the same time and transformative thinking reorders experience, such as creating new forms of object relatedness and greater vitality. EI invites both types of thinking-feeling. In working the composite, Narandja was able to enter multiple perspectives, the three safe images and the one traumatic one, and view them simultaneously. This created a new way to order her experience. As a result, new meaning and aliveness may be generated.

The companionable analyst

In many cases, I have also had success in trauma cases using what Grossmark (2012, p. 630) refers to as "companioning analytic engagement" coupled with judicious interpretations. This dual approach helps generate conditions that spark the patient's imagination.

In companionable listening, the analyst assumes an unobtrusive stance while remaining deeply engaged. Building on the work of the British Independent analysts, particularly Enid and Michael Balint, Grossmark formulates a concept of regression which encompasses "benign regressive mutual regulation" (Grossmark, 2012, p. 629) that helps facilitate trust and entrance into transitional space. The analyst becomes the analyst the patient needs and slowly gains access to unformulated states.

It is noteworthy that although EI is a technique in which the patient is definitely guided in the process, it is also very much remains with the patient's experience, in line with Grossmark's approach. In fact, when the therapist works the dream, he usually does not introduce his own words but rather uses only the words the patient provides, allowing the imagination of the patient to unfold without impingement. In addition, both the patient and therapist are in a hypnogogic state or reverie, similar to Ogden's recommendation that the analyst's participation in the patient's dreaming takes the form of reverie (Ogden, 2004).

Grossmark's position is counter to aspects of the contemporary relational approach, which stress analysis of the intersubjective field, including the effect of the analyst and patient on each other and open expression of countertransference feelings. Some patients find this approach uncomfortable, jarring, or even overwhelming. In instances of trauma, too much introduction of the analyst's feelings and/or the patient's effect on the analyst can be retraumatizing while the unobtrusive approach can be soothing and regulating. Again, each case must be analyzed carefully and worked with accordingly.

Of Italian descent, 45-year-old Diane is at present an increasingly accomplished artist. She had a chaotic and lonely childhood with significant relational trauma. Remembering instances of traumatic interactions, including intense verbal harangues, Diane described her mother as unpredictable and angry and her father as cold and punishing. Her mother was both a talented writer and visual artist. Feeling abandoned when her mother engaged in creative pursuits, her father actively blocked her mother's creative efforts. In his view, these activities took her away from attending to him. Her mother acquiesced but became increasingly angry and resentful.

Artistically creative in multiple areas, Diane chose painting as her focus. Despite innate talent and excellent training, she had great difficulty working. When she would try to paint, she was plagued with traumatic memories and became agitated and panicked. This is in line with Paula Thomson (2002, 2003) who states that when one attempts to create, cortical inhibitory controls are lessened, and traumatic memories can resurface.

Diane and I worked together steadily and slowly, "moving along" in a shared implicit relationship (Stern et al., 1998, p. 903). My unobtrusive, empathic stance helped usher us into transitional space, creating an arena for imagination to develop. Diane became more regulated and her self-states less rigid, creating more fluidity of boundaries both within Diane and between Diane and me, allowing for more therapeutic intimacy. Feeling safer, Diane became more flexible, exploratory and playful – crucial ingredients of the imagination.

At the same time, I was also able to actively discuss and interpret her panic, especially in becoming more creative. When Diane would take a step forward in developing her creativity, she would frequently become acutely anxious and regress to a self-punishing stance. She was very frightened of emerging out of the traumatic matrix of her family structure, which did not permit individuation. She also felt intense guilt about "leaving" her family. For Diane, having a separate life was treasonous. I actively interpreted these dynamics, which helped counter her repetition compulsion and reduce her fears about separation. We also worked many of her dreams together using the EI approach. She felt freer to pursue her art, even using some of the dream imagery in her painting as she directly addressed traumatic themes.

Gradually, she began to overcome her terror of creating. She developed, deepened and expanded her skills. She started to exhibit her work, eventually enjoying a local reputation as a painter. Poetically speaking, Diane was able to dream herself "more fully into existence" (Ogden, 2004, p. 857), something her mother had not been able to do.

Her painting, in turn, is itself therapeutic. It helps aesthetically reframe her trauma, giving her a sense of control and perspective. She can introduce new elements into her experience and therefore continue to recontextualize. In addition, the two-pronged approach of therapeutic companionable listening with judicious interpretations introduces new elements. The therapist is an empathic, knowledgeable presence (as opposed to creating relational trauma) and gradually offers insights that help move the patient along (instead of, for example, the chaotic and/or cold communication to which Diane was exposed in her family of origin).

I tried to navigate a path for Diane that would allow her to separate from her fixed repetitious entanglements and thereby find space to create. A more active relational approach could have been traumatizing, as her mother was eruptive and intrusive. As Grossmark observes, we are always in an intersubjective matrix, but that doesn't mean we have to state this or actively explore our feelings with the patient. A neutral approach would also have been very disturbing, as she experienced a cold, withholding father.

Metaphor and imagination

A flexible use of metaphor is foundational to a healthy imagination. In part, this means that when we experience something in the present, we are able to acknowledge the play of similarity and difference with the past. Modell (2009, p. 6) suggests our early memories are linked to consciousness through metaphor, which "unconsciously categorizes emotional experience establishing similarities and differences between the past and the present." In normal development, as we mature, this unconscious autobiographical memory is constantly being recontextualized or reinterpreted based on current circumstances. Although an event in the present may echo a traumatic childhood memory, we are able to see that the current circumstance is, in fact, quite different and may even be an opportunity for a new experience. We are able to see the similarity but also the difference. This is what is meant by an open and fluid use of metaphor, giving us the ability to process trauma and learn from experience (Modell, 2006).

However, as Modell indicates, in many instances, trauma degrades the metaphoric process, creating an inflexible and foreclosed use of metaphor. The patient interprets the present *only* in terms of the past and becomes mired in the repetition compulsion, as was the case with Diane. There is a compulsive craving to find what one already "knows," making it difficult to learn or experience anything new. Clinicians work to restore a healthy imagination, which will help mitigate future instances of retraumatization and the return of the repetition compulsion.

While traumatized individuals frequently suffer from rigidity of thinking, creative individuals, on the other hand, can tolerate the tension of simultaneous and often opposite views, which requires great emotional stamina and affect regulation. Uncertainty and ambiguity are stressful and difficult. Albert Rothenberg (1990) has named this phenomenon the Janusian process, after the two-headed god Janus standing on a threshold gazing simultaneously in two directions. This Janusian process is more possible if the artist can explore and make a smooth transition among various, sometimes opposing, self-states, as described by Bromberg (2013). EI develops this skill, and Diane benefited from this aspect of the dreamwork.

The infinite 45 minutes: Freud and Margarethe

In a highly imaginative encounter, Freud consulted with 18-year-old Margarethe Lutz in 1936 for one 45-minute session. Margarethe, who had experienced significant relationship trauma, repeatedly said this one session changed her life (Slavin & Rahmani, 2016).

Margarethe was referred to Freud by her family physician who had told her father there was nothing physically wrong with her; rather, she had an illness of the soul. Margarethe had traumatically lost her mother at birth. At the time of the meeting with Freud, she was isolated and depressed, living under the domination of a constricting father. She remarked unhappily that up until this point, "... everything that happened to me was decided behind my back and without my consent" (as quoted in Roos, 2016, p. 295). In a sad revelation, Margarethe said that when she would cry or scream, her father would push her under the bed.

Using both empathy and authority, Freud rekindled her imagination and propelled her forward. Initially, she and her father were in the session. Freud immediately took command, sitting equidistant between Margarethe and her father, as if to indicate they are both important. However, when her father began answering Freud's questions to Margarethe, Freud sent the father out of the room, explaining he wished to talk alone with his patient. He then said to her, "Now it is just the two of us" (as quoted in Roos, 2016, p. 296). He gave Margarethe "advice" – to sit for the end of the love scene in a movie (her father always made her leave before the end to "protect" her from the love scene), to go to dance class and to ski. These were all things Margarethe had told Freud she wanted to do. This kind of advice is basically telling the patient to live her authentic life, which is pretty good advice! And it was accompanied by his empathic gaze and apparent deep interest in her.

Margarethe explains that Freud said:

> 'Being an adult means overcoming complaints and asserting what it means to be a person. Having desires. Contemplating dissent. Asking why things are as they are and not simply accepting everything in silence. Asserting with determination, firmness, and calm what one considers truly important.' And, he prescribed in no uncertain terms, 'the next time there's a kissing scene in a movie, you stay seated!' I am telling you, 'You stay seated!' Pause. Deep eyes. Finally, 'Have me in mind!'
>
> (as quoted in Roos, 2016, p. 297)

Margarethe's father was a powerful and domineering man. Freud's power may have been needed to provide a counterbalancing effect. Margarethe also deeply responded to Freud's empathy. She described how Freud was the first person in her life who really listened. "His whole person was interested in me – and he thus opened something within me that no one else wanted to have opened." Her ever-present desire to reveal herself to another person was "marvelously fulfilled" (as quoted in Roos, 2016, p. 296).

The importance of the paradox of Freud's powerful use of his own authority while at the same time allowing Margarethe to have her authority (for the first time in her life) is discussed by Jonathan Slavin (2016). He asserts that maintaining this paradox gives both patient and therapist the opportunity to have a "say." Freud was a figure of great authority and expressed that; however, he also saw Margarethe's uniqueness and facilitated her wish to be born as a person.

This session has aspects of Baumrind's (1966) authoritative parenting style, a flexible blend of authority and freedom, characterized by warmth and moderate control (with the reasons for the rules frequently explained). Giving enough space for imagination but enough structure for security and self-regulation, this approach has been positively associated with creativity (Miller & Gerald, 1979; Parcheh Baf, 1990; Mouchiroud & Bernoussi, 2008; Fearon et al., 2013; Heo, 2014; Mozafari, 2014; Mehrinejad et al., 2015). Structure combined with empathy gives the child a safe space in which to imagine. I see a parallel in my treatment of Diane. The unobtrusive stance represents the empathy while the interpretations represent authority, together creating the space to imagine.

Margarethe felt secure in the firm structure set by Freud (his authority in sending her father out, in telling her to sit down for the whole movie, etc.) while she also enjoyed space for exploration of her own wishes and thoughts (how Freud listened carefully and gazed at her with empathy, encouraging the expression of her own desires). As Baumrind might have predicted, Margarethe did develop creatively. In addition to becoming a wife and mother, she had a successful career as a sculptor.

Similarly, I want clinicians to find their own power and individuality and help their patients do so as well. While clinicians need to study widely and learn from "authorities," each must also find the space to explore and discover his or her own viewpoint. To do so, one needs free access to imagination.

Loss of the empathic other

Freud's treatment of Margarethe, as well as my work with Diane, can be viewed as a restoration of the loss of the empathic other. Laub (2005) writes brilliantly about this type of loss in Holocaust victims.[2] In many instances, the inner connection to the good object is lost, damaging the ability to symbolize and shattering the imagination. The victim can no longer create an authentic narrative or find meaning in experience. Although the example of Margarethe or Diane is certainly not in this extreme category, similar principles apply. The traumatized patient needs a therapeutic holding environment to construct a new narrative and restore a sense of connection and flexibility of imaginative feeling and thought.

In addition to rebuilding the link between self and other, Dori Laub and Nanette Auerhahn (1989) recommend that the therapist do more integrative work than is usual. This helps construct a meaningful narrative for the traumatized patient. Freud provided much integrative work with Margarethe, as I did with Diane. Finally, especially during affect storms of the patient, Laub and Auerhahn write that the therapist cannot maintain a therapeutically neutral stance, as this may exacerbate the patient's periodic feelings of terror and be experienced as a denial of suffering. Freud's work with Margarethe was affirmatively pro-growth and not neutral.

Many traumatized patients no longer feel at home in the world yet also have lost a sense of desire to seek home (comfort), as in the extreme withdrawal of the Cat Dreamer. Judith Brisman (2002) writes it is the intolerance of wanting that shuts down human growth and thwarts therapeutic progress. Adam Phillips (2000) states that needs and wants develop in an interpersonal context, which can give shape to the more formless experience of desire. In psychotherapy therapists work to contain the trauma so desire and agency can emerge. Diane was able once again to create. Similarly, the Cat Dreamer began to communicate and cooperate with treatment.

The neuropsychology of trauma

Exploring imagination developmentally helps us understand more deeply the difficulties caused by trauma, which negatively alter the maturation of the child's right brain. Conversely, it is the sensitive, caring relationship with caretakers that facilitate the positive emergence of the right hemisphere (RH) and accompanying imaginative facility in the young child.

While creativity involves both right and left-brain operations, the role of the RH is essential to the development of healthy imagination, the foundation of which is metaphor, as discussed above. Marks-Tarlow (2012) addresses how metaphor arises primarily from the divergent and synthetic processing of the RH and cites Schore who "... views imagery, symbolic thought, and the visual imagination, all so prevalent in metaphor, to represent the apex of 'high right' functioning" (Marks-Tarlow, 2012, p. 162).

Developmentally our first metaphors emerge concretely through the body when the RH is developing (Modell, 2006). The right is more closely connected to the body than the later developing left hemisphere (LH) (Modell, 2006). Children commonly use gestures and bodily actions to describe metaphorical events, such as a four-year-old crawling on all fours when asked how time crawls (Ozcaliskan, 2007). Later, instead of whole-body enactments, children begin to produce metaphorical hand gestures that convey information. A toddler may use space metaphorically, using nearness to his body to mean similar and farness to mean dissimilar (Thelen & Smith, 1994).

The RH is primed for creative thinking and therefore the possibility of change. More capable of a frame shift, the RH is especially important for flexibility of thought. The unfamiliar activates the right; it thrives in ambiguity while embracing the novelty of the moment. Once a phrase has become old or clichéd, it will move into left side for processing (McGilchrist, 2009). Regarding problem solving, the RH presents an array of possible solutions, which remain alive while alternatives are explored. The left, by contrast, takes the single solution that seems best to fit what it already knows and latches onto it.

Intimately connected with the limbic system, an ancient subcortical system that is involved in the experience of emotion, the RH is also essential to emotional understanding and regulation. Specializing in nonverbal communication and the implicit, the RH helps us empathize (Graham, 2004), perhaps even "read each other's minds," contributing to the relational imagination.

For all these reasons and more, Schore (2011, 2014) writes that psychotherapy is right-brain to right-brain communication, that is, first and foremost, the therapist and patient are relating to each other emotionally, not analytically or intellectually. Therapy is attachment based and aimed at reactivating and rewiring early unconscious dysfunctional patterns stored in the RH. The therapist slowly helps the patient regulate affect and develop empathy as well as resilience. This may include working with intense enactments as well as playful and nonverbal unconscious communication between patient and therapist, as a mother might with a young child. Most patients come to us with emotional disturbances, and therapy, in part, serves as rehabilitation of disrupted right brain functioning.

Trauma disrupts the ability to play, a precursor to imaginative and creative thinking (Schore, 2001). In early trauma affecting the RH, the primitive defense of dissociation develops and more complex defenses fail to organize. The child cannot move flexibly between a resting quiet state (inhibitory) to a more active state (excitatory). Unless the child can do this, he cannot be involved in dyadic play with its interactively created high levels of arousal. The inability to engage in interactive play, in children or adults, is an indicator of disturbance and is reminiscent of the lack of flexibility in states of trauma, as discussed by Modell. Helping the patient recover this capacity is an important ingredient in healing. Winnicott (1971) famously wrote that if the patient cannot play, then this must be the first order of treatment. It is in playing that the patient is creative, and in being creative, the patient discovers his true self. Winnicott locates play in the potential space between mother and baby. When the infant/caretaker relationship is good, this enables the emergence of potential or transitional space. Similarly, the if the therapeutic dyad is functioning well, the patient is ushered into potential space where play becomes possible.

The art of survival

While in many cases trauma disturbs the imagination, there are cases of amazing resilience and imaginative agency in the face of trauma. Laub and Podell (1995) discuss Helen K, a Holocaust survivor who recounts how her 13-year-old brother suffocated in an overcrowded transport wagon and died in her arms. At the moment of his death, she vowed, "I'm going to live." She testifies, "I said to myself, I want to live one day after Hitler, one day after the end of the war" (as quoted in Laub & Podell, 1995, p. 999).

Through this imaginative act, she grasped her connection to life. With courageous defiance, she was able to survive the camps in the face of physical deterioration. She states, "After I was liberated … a Russian doctor examined me and said, 'Under normal circumstances you would not have survived …. It's just a medical miracle that you survived'" (as quoted in Laub & Podell, 1995, p. 999).

Somehow this teenage girl maintained a belief that gave meaning to the unimaginable cruelty that surrounded her. In her belief that she will outlive

Hitler, she accurately understood and defied Hitler's dictum, that each Jew is worthless and deserves to die. She found self-respect and meaning in her wish to survive. She was able to recontextualize her experience and not become a victim. Therapists attempt to help patients develop the resilience and strength that Helen K was miraculously able to do on her own.

Helen K's response is termed the "art of trauma" by Laub and Podell (2005, p. 991). This includes the creation of traditional forms of art such as literature, music and sculpture in response to trauma as well as imaginative acts that occur spontaneously within the process of survival. The authors indicate ... "that survival itself should be considered as a type of art of trauma when it is made possible by a creative comprehension of reality analogous to that which characterizes more conventional forms of the art of trauma" (Laub & Podell, 2005, p. 991).

The value of the art of trauma is in its ability to engender meaning (Laub & Podell, 1995; Rose, 1996). Through dialogue in the present, art revisits the hidden past of trauma. As a holding, witnessing "other," it validates the reality of the traumatic event while providing a presence that begins to restore the loss of the internal empathic other. Giving form to chaos, it also helps the artist gain perspective and strength. Indirectly, other trauma victims who view such work come to know their own trauma as well. According to Laub and Podell, the art of trauma may be the only means to adequately depict extreme trauma.

Personal example

In an attempt to find new approaches to grapple with trauma as well as benefit from the therapeutic effect of the "art of trauma," I have embarked on writing a series of plays (Domash, 2015, 2017, 2018; Domash & Rappoport, 2016). Wrestling with themes of freedom and abuse, the plays pose the question: How can one emerge from the confines of trauma and find the courage to change? The plays have been performed for audiences of psychotherapists and patients as well as the general public and have been used for clinical training purposes. After each performance, we have a "talk back," an audience discussion led by skilled drama therapist Jarred Sharar.

Although meant to be entertainment, the plays and "talk backs" are potentially therapeutic, providing a holding environment and reestablishing the sense of an "empathic other," creating a dialogue in the present. They offer the audience safe aesthetic distance so, if relevant, audience members can identify with a traumatized character or situation without becoming overwhelmed (Landy, 1983) and begin to consider new perspectives offered in the production.

One of my plays, *A Joke for Bella,* tells the story of the friendship between two women in a work camp in World War II. Providing a witnessing presence for each other, the two women use humor and fantasy to the point of delusion to cope with the stress. All the jokes in the play are authentic and from records of jokes told in the camps. The play models possibilities for resilience and strength through the comfort and containment of friendship.

My own history includes great aunts and uncles living in Europe who were taken to the camps. Some survived, and this play could be their story, while others perished. Although living in the United states, my grandmother and mother suffered great anguish as a result of what happened to their extended family in Europe. In creating this play, I felt some healing in them (and in me who witnessed their suffering), even though they passed away many years ago.

It is interesting that in the "talk back" after one of the performances, an audience member strongly objected to our beginning the audience discussion so quickly after the play ended. She felt we needed time to experience silent, empty space to grasp the terror in the play. Similarly, Laub and Podell (1995) stress the need for omissions and silences in the art of trauma. For example, breaks in poetry or holes in a canvas can enable the reader to the experience the black void present in trauma. From the darkness, as Kabbalah professes, new possibilities emerge. The trauma is remembered, and healing can begin.

Trauma and the struggle to create

While there can be amazing resilience in trauma victims, many traumatized artists struggle with the creative process. Thomson, a creativity researcher, dancer and choreographer, broadly divides the creative process into two phases: inspiration and elaboration. In this first phase, there is reduced cortical activity, creating less inhibition of disturbing memories. This can frighten a traumatized artist because the controls to suppress the trauma loosen and traumatic memories can surface, evoking terrifying feelings of disintegration (Thomson, 2003). This may help explain why many of the artists who attempted to deal with the Holocaust were eventually overcome with despair and committed suicide (Laub and Podell, 1995). Short of the desperate act of suicide, fantasy may be deployed as a means of dissociative escape. This repeated withdrawal leads to further reduction in the range and depth of creative expression necessary for mature artistic work (Thomson, 2002).

As suggested above, creativity and trauma (pathological dissociation) can involve similar brain areas (Irwin, 2001; Watson, 2001; Dorahy, 2002). The creative process and dissociation often involve states similar to déjà vu, trance states, out-of-body experiences and mystical moments, all of which involve decreased frontal arousal.

Creative individuals are novelty and stimulus seeking, which includes fantasy proneness; fantasy proneness has also been strongly correlated to dissociation (Pekala et al., 2000; Somer & Orit, 2001). Fantasy proneness refers to a small group of people who are often absorbed in fantasy, report vivid childhood memories, experience strong bodily concomitants of fantasies and have out-of-body and other paranormal experiences as well as intense religious experiences (Wilson & Barber, 1983).

It is at first confusing that creative people and some highly disturbed people may both use dissociation. However, Thomson et al. (2009) write we may need to more clearly differentiate between creative and pathological states. Depending on other factors, dissociation can be pathological or non-pathological. Artists in creative states may be biased toward enhanced dissociative states, such as absorption, imagination and identity diffusion. If this dissociation is coupled with good affect control (so that the dissociative state can be flexibly moved in and out of), the creative process is facilitated, and the dissociation is not pathological. Similarly, successful artists are able to use their fantasy proneness to support their art just as the characters in my play were able to use fantasy, even delusion, to successfully withstand the trauma of the work camp.

Many studies demonstrate neuronal damage associated with trauma and dissociation (Thomson, 2002). A few of many examples are damage to the hippocampal and parahippocampal regions, areas critical for creativity. Studies have shown that decreased volume in these areas is linked to trauma and dissociation. Damage to the hippocampal area, in particular, causes disruptions in autobiographical memory formation. This directly impacts working memory and the fluency of associational memory, both necessary for creativity (Thomson, 2002).

The creative individual with a trauma history is aware of these problems and can become profoundly frustrated over the inability to fluently associate and freely engage in sustained divergent thought.[3] While creativity can heal many emotional wounds, the damage that occurs during prolonged periods of trauma may be so great as to be irremediable. Patrick Bissell, an acclaimed ballet dancer, was reportedly physically and emotionally abused by his mother. He told an interviewer "I do good performances and then I punish myself with drugs. I try to destroy myself. It's a weird kind of cycle" (as quoted in Thomson, 2002, p. 11). He died shortly after this from an overdose. Tragically, his creativity could not sustain him.

The therapeutic goal with all patients, and trauma patients in particular, is to transform repetitive, stereotyped ways of thinking/feeling into flexible modes to facilitate new ways of being in this world. Ogden (2004) writes we help our patients dream their interrupted and undreamt dreams. I say that, additionally, we can help patients enter and embody the images in their dreams, whether the images are parts of the self or new subjectivities entirely, so they can expand their imagination and become who they are meant to be.

Notes

1 The *treatment* of trauma is a vast subject. There are myriad degrees and varieties of trauma and many specific treatments available. A thorough discussion of this is beyond the scope of this chapter. This chapter is limited to the disruptive effect of trauma on the imagination.

2 Holocaust victims experienced trauma on a scale almost unimaginable and differ from other trauma victims in the *depth* and scope of their suffering.

Nevertheless, we can learn from research regarding the Holocaust and apply these principles to much lesser, although significant, relational trauma.

3 Divergent thinking is a process of generating creative ideas in a spontaneous, nonlinear fashion in order to solve a problem. It *expands outward* to come up with unique ideas. Convergent thinking, the opposite, is systematic and logical and *narrows down* multiple ideas to obtain a correct answer, as on a multiple-choice test.

References

Baumrind, D. (1966). Effects of authoritative parental control on child behavior. *Child Development*, 37(4):887–907.

Bosnak, R. (2008). *Embodiment: Creative imagination in medicine, art and travel.* New York: Routledge.

Brisman, J. (2002). Wanting. *Contemporary Psychoanalysis*, 38(2):329–343.

Bromberg, P.M. (2013). Hidden in plain sight: Thoughts on imagination and the lived unconscious. *Psychoanalytic Dialogues*, 23:1–14.

Domash, L. (2015). *The Meeting of My Dreams* (theatrical presentation). Performances: April 26, 2015, 35th Annual Spring Meeting of the Division of Psychoanalysis (39) of the American Psychological Association, *Life in Psychoanalysis in Life*; July 19, 2015, Society for Exploration of Psychoanalytic Therapies and Theology, Allentown, PA.

Domash, L. (2017). *A Joke for Bella* (theatrical presentation). Performances: March 22, 2017, TBG Studio Theatre, 312 West 36th Street, New York; April 21, 2017, New York University, 35 West 4th Street, New York; April 30, 2017, Jewish Enrichment Center, 38 West 13th Street, New York.

Domash, L. (2018). *Living on the Edge: A Magical Mixture of the Sacred and Profane* (theatrical presentation). Performances: April 23, 2018, TBG Studio Theatre, 312 West 36th Street, New York; April 24 and 25, Jewish Enrichment Center, 38 West 13th Street, New York.

Domash, L. & Rappoport, E. (2016). *When Alice Meets Eve in the Gardens of the Known and Unknown* (theatrical presentation). Performances: May 8, 2016, Branded Saloon, 603 Vanderbilt Avenue, Brooklyn, NY; June 4, 2016, New York Psychological Association Convention: Advancing the Practice of Psychology: Ethics, Risk Management and Innovative Methods, White Plains, NY; October 8, 2016, *Seeing Red Conference: Exploring the archetypal roots of feminine oppression through a deep engagement of the analytic and artistic*, Assisi Institute, Stonington, CT.

Dorahy, M.J. (2002). Cognitive inhibition in dissociative identity disorder: Developing an understanding of working memory function in DID. *Journal of Trauma and Dissociation*, 3(3):111–132.

Fearon, D., Copeland, D. & Saxon, T. (2013). The relationship between parenting styles and creativity in a sample of Jamaican children. *Creativity Research Journal*, 251:119–128.

Graham, L. (2004). https://lindagraham-mft.net/right-brain-to-right-brain-therapy

Grossmark, R. (2012). The unobtrusive relational analyst. *Psychoanalytic Dialogues*, 22:629–646.

Hartmann, E. (2001). *Dreams and nightmares: The origin and meaning of dreams.* New York: Perseus Publishing.

Heo, N. (2014). The relationship between creative potential and self-regulation among high achieving young adults with the moderating effects of parenting styles. PhD (Doctor of Philosophy) thesis, University of Iowa. http://ir.uiowa.edu/etd/4643

Irwin, H.J. (2001). The relationship between dissociative tendencies and schizotypy: An artifact of childhood trauma? *Journal of Clinical Psychology*, 57(3):331–342.

Landy, R. (1983). The use of distancing in drama therapy. *The Arts in Psychotherapy*, 10:175–185.

Laub, D. (2005). Traumatic shutdown of narrative and symbolization. *Contemporary Psychoanalysis*, 41(2):307–326.

Laub, D. & Auerhahn, N.C. (1989). Failed empathy – A central theme in the survivor's Holocaust experience. *Psychoanalytic Psychology*, 6(4):377–400.

Laub, D. & Podell, D. (1995). Art and trauma. *International Journal of Psychoanalysis*, 76:991–1005.

Marks-Tarlow, T. (2012). *Clinical intuition in psychotherapy*. New York: Norton.

Mehrinejad, S.A., Rajabimoghadamb, S. & Tarsafic, M. (May 14–16, 2015). The relationship between parenting styles and creativity and the predictability of creativity by parenting styles. 6th World conference on Psychology Counseling and Guidance, Antalya, Turkey.

Miller, B.C. & Gerard, D. (1979). Family influence on the development of creativity in children: An integrative review. *The Family Coordinator*, 28(3):295–312.

Modell, A. (2006). *Imagination and the meaningful brain*. Cambridge, MA: MIT Press.

Modell, A. (2009). Metaphor – The bridge between feelings and knowledge. *Psychoanalytic Inquiry*, 29:6–11.

Mouchiroud, C. & Bernoussi, A (2008). An empirical study of the construct validity of social creativity. *Learning and Individual Differences*, 18(4):372–380.

Mozafari, S. (2014). Prediction of creativity and academic achievement based on child rearing styles. *International Journal of Psychology and Behavioral Research*, 33(3):166–176.

Ogden, T.H. (2004). This art of psychoanalysis: Dreaming undreamt dreams and interrupted cries. *International Journal of Psychoanalysis*, 85(4):857–877.

Ogden, T.H. (2010). On three forms of thinking: Magical thinking, dream thinking, and transformative thinking. *Psychoanalytic Quarterly*, 79(2):317–347.

Ozcaliskan, S. (2007). Metaphors we move by: Children's developing understanding of motion in typologically distinct languages. *Metaphor and Symbol*, 22(2):147–168.

Parcheh Baf, D. (1990). Creativity in genius students. MA thesis. Islamic Azad University.

Pekala, R.J., Kumar, V.K., Ainslie, G., Elliott, N.C., Mullen, K.J., Salinger, M.M. & Masten, E. (1999–2000). Dissociation as a functioning of child abuse and fantasy-proneness in a substance abuse population. *Imagination, Cognition and Personality*, 19(2):105–129.

Phillips, A. (May 12–13, 2000). On what we need: A celebration of Mannie Ghent. Presented at a multimedia conference celebrating the life and work of Emmanuel Ghent, New York University Postdoctoral Program in Psychotherapy and Psychoanalysis, New York City, NY.

Roos, P. (2016). The great listener. *Psychoanalytic Perspectives*, 13(3):294–299.
Rose, G.J. (1996). *Necessary illusion: Art as 'witness'*. New York: International Universities Press.
Rothenberg, A. (1990). *Creativity and madness: New findings and old stereotypes*. Baltimore, MD: The John Hopkins University Press.
Schore, A.N. (2001). The effects of early relational trauma on right brain development, affect regulation and infant mental health. *Infant Mental Health Journal*, 22(1–2):201–269.
Schore, A.N. (2011). The right brain implicit self lies at the core of psychoanalytic psychotherapy. *Psychoanalytic Dialogues*, 21:75–100.
Schore, A.N. (2014). The right brain is dominant in psychotherapy. *Psychotherapy*, 51(3):388–397.
Slavin, J.H. (2016). "I never felt I should think about Freud": From authority to liberation in psychoanalytic work. *Psychoanalytic Perspectives*, 13(3):321–325.
Slavin, J.H. & Rahmani, M. (2016). Those 45 minutes changed my life: The Meeting of Sigmund Freud and Margarethe Lutz. *Psychoanalytic Perspectives*, 13(3):291–293.
Somer, E. & Orit, N. (2000–2001). An ethnographic study of former DID patients. *Imagination, Cognition and Personality*, 20:315–346.
Stern, D.N., Sander, L., Nahum, J., Harrison, A., Lyons-Ruth, K., Morgan, A., Bruschweiler-Stern, N. & Tronick, E. (1998). Noninterpretive mechanisms in psychoanalytic therapy: The "something more" than interpretation. *International Journal of Psycho-Analysis*, 79:903–921.
Thelen, E. & Smith, L. (1994). *A dynamic systems approach to the development of cognition and action*. Cambridge, MA: MIT Press.
Thomson, P. (November 11, 2002). The traumatized imagination: Creativity, trauma and the neurobiology of the resilient spirit. 19th ISSD Conference (International Society for the Study of Trauma and Dissociation), Baltimore, MD. www.healingresources.info/article_thomson1.htm.
Thomson, P. (May 17–18, 2003). From neurons to neighborhoods: New ways to prevent and heal emotional trauma in children and adults. Second Annual Conference, Los Angeles, CA. Interview with Paula Thomson, PsyD by M. Winchester.
Thomson, P., Keehn, E.B. & Gumpel, T. (2009). Generators and interpreters in a performing arts population: Dissociation, trauma, fantasy proneness, and affective states. *Creativity Research Journal*, 21(1):72–91.
Watson, D. (2001). Dissociations of the night: Individual differences in sleep-related experiences and their relation to dissociation and schizotypy. *Journal of Abnormal Psychology*, 110:526–535.
Wilson, S.C. & Barber, T.X. (1983). The fantasy-prone personality: Implications for understanding imagery, hypnosis and parapsychological phenomena. In A.A. Sheikh (Ed.), *Imagery: Current theory, research and application* (pp. 340–387). New York: John Wiley & Sons.
Winnicott, D.W. (1971). *Playing and reality*. London: Tavistock Publications.

Chapter 8

How art heals[1]

The aesthetic imagination heals. Instead of merely expressing the self, the artist reshapes it. She brings her unconscious thoughts and feelings into the external world and in so doing transforms them (Bollas, 2011a). As we view or read or listen to a work of art, we participate in this transformation.

The transformative process is an interdependence of fragmentation and integration. To formulate something new, old structures must be broken down. Then the artist reintegrates these fragments into a new construction. Referring to Kleinian theory, Bion sees growth and the creative process as a dialectic between the paranoid-schizoid and depressive position[2] (Glover, 2009). The artist may experience feelings of fragmentation (a move toward the paranoid schizoid position), a crisis of sorts, as she works on her art. Then she may move toward feelings of greater integration (the depressive position), as she transforms the fragmented pieces into aesthetic wholes. These movements echo the psychotherapy process, which repeatedly moves between conflict/regression and creation/resolution. The patient may have to tolerate feelings of confusion and emptiness in order to work toward re-integration and creation.

In part, it is the transformative power of art that makes it so appealing. We may underestimate the nearly universal need for transformational experiences (Bollas, 2011b). The mother is soothing to the infant but more importantly, transformative. The unarticulated memory trace of this experience remains alive forever, and the wish for deeply mutative experiences reoccurs throughout life. The adult's feeling of being held by a poem, a painting or a piece of writing harkens back to this (Bollas, 1978). Such moments feel familiar, uncanny and outside cognitive coherence. Growing out of the potential (transitional) play space between infant and caretaker, these cultural, aesthetic experiences occur in the potential space between the individual and his environment (Winnicott, 1971). It is here in this scared space that the individual experiences creative living.

This chapter explores many art forms as examples of areas of play that can usher patients into imaginal, potential space, providing the safety to explore conflict and/or trauma and the opportunity to experience transformation. As discussed in Chapter 7, trauma patients in particular can benefit from therapeutic exploration in the arts, allowing them to represent trauma as well as introduce new elements into their experience, achieving a sense of mastery. In fact, Laub and Podell (1995) suggest that the "art of trauma," defined as artwork that deals with trauma as well as spontaneous acts of survival, may be the only effective way to represent trauma.

Language and poetic psychoanalysis

While therapists certainly cannot expect to reach the genius of a poet or novelist in their use of words, language – including feeling-tone, sense of aliveness, nuance, voice and musicality – is crucial to the success of the work. With our language-relationship we encourage the patient to speak more freely. Both sides of the therapeutic dyad become more aware of unconscious patterns, and meaning begins to appear.

Exquisitely attuned to the notion of "voice" in psychoanalysis, Ogden (1998, p. 426) writes, "Creating a voice with which to speak or to write might be thought of as a way, perhaps the principal way, in which individuals bring themselves into being, come to life, through their use of language." "Voice" is the distinctive way each member of the dyad sounds as he or she communicates.

The voice of the patient and analyst are separate and distinct yet both come from the shared unconscious space of the dyad, creating the "analytic third" (Ogden, 1994, 1998). Listening carefully to his own voice and to the voice of the patient, Ogden asks if either or both voices are deadened. If so, this alerts him to a stagnant phase of the therapy; it is the aliveness of the voice that matters most to Ogden.

Ogden describes how the analyst creates a new voice at the start of each therapy, even in each encounter, not knowing how it may develop as the therapy evolves. He comments:

> As many times as I have entered into an analytic experience with a new patient over the past twenty-five years, I am each time surprised by the fact that I speak with a different voice (more accurately, a different set of voices in continual transition) with each new patient. I do not and could not preconceive the voices with which I will hear myself speaking. For me, this is one of the wonders of spending one's life in the practice of psychoanalysis. Not only is my voice different with each patient, when an analysis is going well my voice and that of the patient are developing new 'oversounds' in the course of each analytic hour and during the course of the weeks, months, and years of an analysis.
>
> (Ogden, 1998, p. 446)

This issue of voice is especially interesting to me, as that is how I conceptualized my struggle with writing this book. Can I find my voice, broadly defined as my unique style of language as well as my own point of view? Does my voice have to be consistent or can it change with each chapter, depending on the content? Even as it changes, I still want it to be "mine." I fear being the "dummy" and the "experts" my ventriloquists. My goal has been to give shape to my own voice, for better or worse and not parrot others. Otherwise, why write at all?

Similarly, the therapist wants her patient to find his authentic voice, which will initially evolve into a coconstruction arising from the therapeutic dyad but ultimately the patient leaves treatment with his own voice. In the same way, I have had to blend with the experts but then reemerge with a voice that is mine.

Psychoanalytic psychotherapist Mary Wallach is in search of the poetic analyst. Both the poet and the psychoanalyst must find the words that create an authentic, "transforming truth" (Wallach, 2003, p. 398). The poetic analyst views therapy as a dyadic process which translates the feelings, unconscious fantasies and nonverbal communications occurring in the session into words. The aesthetic pleasure of finding the right words also helps the patient transform his pain. As the dialogue continues, patient and analyst cocreate a body of "blended imaginings" (Wallach, 2003, p. 400), which are all contained in the session. This paradoxically both joins and separates analyst and patient, allowing them to experience their intersubjective truth together and then to separate, as the patient terminates.

The importance of words goes beyond their meaning or even the pleasure of speaking language. Rather, it is how they can contain and integrate the dialectics of conscious and unconscious, implicit and explicit, logical and magical, revealing the essence of the communication between the dyad in a highly focused way (Arieti, 1976). Words are "vital interpersonal currency that, exchanged in exactly the right combination (and, like currency, any number of combinations may be right), promote shared discovery" (Wallach, 2003, p. 407). Through repetition and interpretation, words are given new meaning and gradually, facilitate change.

Therapeutic value of poetry

Poetry can have an impact on mental pain[3] that is akin to a psychoanalytic intervention (Akhtar, 2000). Poetry can facilitate self-reflection and regulation, aid in the mourning process and help the patient accept disavowed parts of the self. In addition, what Salman Akhtar (2000, p. 235) terms the "libidinal aspects of poetic form" – the richness of metaphor, pattern, design, rhythm and meter – facilitates entrance into transitional space and the possibility of creative, healing solutions.

As an example, Ms. K, a highly talented but fragile 25-year-old patient, described her struggle with keeping her sense of creativity and vitality alive, including a flexible use of metaphor, as described by Modell (2006). When she left home for college, early traumatic separation anxieties were triggered. She became so panicked and depressed, she felt she was on the verge of collapse. To combat this, she put up poems all over the walls of her dorm room to articulate how she felt. W.B Yeats' "The Lake Isle of Innisfree" comforted her.[4] The poem had the calming, mesmerizing quality of a lullaby. She was transported to that cabin Yeats described and found some peace there. Gerard Manley Hopkins' "My Own Heart" helped her feel compassion for herself and gently prodded her to more self-care.[5] Emily Dickinson's "Wild Nights! Wild Nights!" allowed her to dream of love and passion.[6] Ms. K identified with Dickinson, especially in her isolation and unfulfilled desires, and this reduced her loneliness. William Carlos Williams' "The Red Wheelbarrow"[7] and e.e. cummings' "I thank You God for most this amazing"[8] roused her to focus on the beauty in everyday life. Williams' poem stunned her in its elegant simplicity, allowing her to pause and focus, while cummings' lush language thrilled her in its intensity. In total, these poems offered comfort and consolation, encouraged understanding and self-acceptance and subtly fostered agency and self-determination. She did not want to lose her imagination. She struggled and succeeded.

I would say to both patient and therapist, read but also write poetry, no matter how clumsy or awkward you may feel, as this can challenge traditional meaning and keep the focus on the music of the patient's words, both of which aid in recognizing underlying patterns and help the patient heal. The curative power of *Wonderland* was definitely in the music of the words, not in the "knowledge" I gained from them. The music inspired me to "know" I could move beyond my current situation and discover something new.

As mentioned, Akhtar (2000) writes about the value of poetry when in psychic pain; it helps the person move away from the agony of present circumstances and quiets troubling inner dialogues. The poetry turns the passive experience of pain into an active, creative experience, which gives the reader hope. If I find a poem that expresses a patient's conflict, I might read it to them or have them read it. An example is "The Journey"[9] by Mary Oliver, which discusses the need to define oneself and move forward with life, although there may be strong forces working against this. I read this to a patient to validate her right to separate from her family, despite intense feelings of guilt. When a patient has made a great deal of progress, I may use a poem to underscore her achievement. A patient was ready to terminate group therapy, and, with another group member, I had her read the poem

"Chrysalis Diary" from *Joyful Noise: Poems for Two Voices.*[10] This poem tells the story of the painful change from moth to butterfly, finally flying free. The poem affirmed and commemorated her therapeutic journey.

Formal poetry therapy has been studied extensively and found to have numerous positive benefits (Heines, 2011). Examples include the abovementioned reduction in mental pain (Akhtar, 2000), lowered anxiety in cancer patients (Tegner et al., 2009) and bereaved patients (O'Conner et al., 2003), improved immune function (Pennebaker et al., 1988) and improved functioning in domestic violence survivors (Dubransky et al., 2019).

The importance of surprise and strangeness

Describing how poems come to him in unexpected moments, the Irish lyric poet Michael Longley (2016) explains how poems "find" him when he is at the butcher shop or the ice cream parlor. Without this element of surprise, he says, his poems would be lifeless. So, too, our therapy. Surprising the patient is an important part of expanding the imagination. In line with Wallach's thinking, whenever possible, if there is a choice about how to phrase something to a patient, I try to word it as surprisingly and poetically as possible, even a little "off-beat." This subtly challenges the patient in her habitual way of thinking and may encourage her to be a little more off "message," a little more audacious. This can facilitate the spontaneous, improvisational thinking needed for fresh approaches.

Some confirming evidence is provided by researchers studying implicit learning. Travis Proulx and Steven Heine (2009) tested whether providing a challenge to meaning (such as, reading an absurdist story which surprises the reader with unexpected and strange connections and illustrations) would cause subjects to more easily learn new patterns – in this particular study, enhanced performance on an artificial grammar learning task. One group read a modified version of Kafka's absurdist short story, *The Country Doctor*, which contained non sequiturs and bizarre illustrations unrelated to the text, and the other group read a story with the same title that followed a conventional narrative. Subjects were then shown a seemingly meaningless string of letters, which actually did conform to an artificial grammar and had hidden patterns.

The results indicated that the group that read the absurdist story were more motivated and more accurate in solving the "problem," that is, finding the underlying patterns in the string of letters, than the group that read the conventional story. The researchers confirmed their hypothesis that the implicit learning of novel associations is enhanced when traditional meaning is challenged beforehand. Absurdist texts may cause a breakdown of expected associations and throw the subject "off balance." This can create an urgency to reestablish a sense of meaning, leading to an "aha" moment.

Under experimental conditions, the subjects exposed to the absurdist story were able to find *or learn* patterns that were hidden but already there. In a sense, patients face the same problem: how to learn new patterns that may already be present, as for example, a patient who continually seeks out hurtful partners resembling her stepmother when she has several other significant kind and supportive family members. What would motivate her to unconsciously learn a new pattern that to date has remained hidden to her? How can the clinician support this? With some patients, therapists may need to introduce the right amount of strangeness in their use of language to help the patient reassemble her thinking to allow innovative solutions – enough dissonance to challenge habitual patterns but not so much as to unmoor the patient.

I can't say it better than the Brazilian writer Clarice Lispector who in her novel Agua Viva, writes "And when I think a word is strange that's where it achieves the meaning. And when I think life is strange that's where life begins" (Lispector, 2012, p. 76). Rafferty in reviewing Lispector's work writes, "Her stories are full of strange words, in strange combinations and, every now and then, the harmony of a new-minted morning" (Rafferty, 2015, p. 1). Would we, with our words, be able to bring the feeling of a new-minted morning to our patients!

In a similar vein, the Surrealist poets and painters stressed the element of surprise and strangeness. Attempting to liberate the imagination and free people from habitual ways of thinking, they embraced idiosyncrasy and juxtaposed images normally not found together to generate emotional power and poetic reality, and, most importantly, to let the unconscious express itself, as therapists aim to do. This contributes to emotional freedom, allowing one to become more whole and independent (Breton, 1969; Pynchon, 1998; Dali, 2007).

The book as psychotherapist/the book as supervisor

Patients frequently report receiving help from reading fiction and nonfiction. An interaction of unconscious forces can develop between the book and the reader. Zelnick (2014) articulates how reading can be an interpersonal experience; the text can "speak" and seem to react in different ways at different times depending on one's state of mind. He gives an example of his surprise in reading a familiar biblical text when he suddenly saw something he had not seen before. As a result, he was shocked into considering some unfamiliar ideas and feelings about himself. Aware of the tension between familiarity and surprise, he suggests that he saw the new aspect of the text only when he was emotionally prepared to notice. He then makes connections between his reaction to the text and the kind of dramatic surprise that can occur in therapy. Either patient or therapist can notice something different about himself or the other, and psychological shifts can occur. In another vein, Bollas (2011b) discusses how literature can be transformative when the reader experiences intense rapport with a text that evokes a sense memory of being with the original caretaker, experienced as a transformational object. This is often felt to be uncanny or mystical.

As I described in Chapter 1, as a young reader of seven or eight, I had a therapeutic experience with *Alice's Adventures in Wonderland* (Carroll & Gardner, 2000). Carroll's creation is a dream turned into a poem turned into a fairy tale, and it changed me. As a dream-poem, it has the potential to help access the unconscious, contain fears and inspire creativity. It appeals to all ages. Virginia Woolf went so far as to say that the Alice books are not "books for children. They are the only books in which we become children" (Woolf, 1971, p. 48).

I read *Wonderland* countless times, feeling very connected to Alice. She was very much a "participant" in this process. I "listened" to Alice, as if she could speak. We spoke to each other with our own voices but eventually, after many, many readings, from a common area of jointly constructed unconscious experience, generating what Ogden (1994, 1998) calls the "analytic third."

This helped me "know" I could move beyond my current situation of being a "good girl." It was an antidote to my literal understanding of my family's practice of Orthodox Judaism, including the multiple rules I imposed on myself and to the ubiquitous conservatism of the small Pennsylvanian town in which I lived. Looking back, I wanted more freedom but didn't dare take it. Alice helped me become less repressed, like "literary play therapy."

Turning rules upside down, Carroll's fiction reveals their, at times, ludicrous foundations. Carroll portrays the futility and absurdity of the White Rabbit, who is consumed by time but seems to get nowhere, and the Mad Hatter, who has tea every day, all day, as time is standing still at 6 PM (tea time). In the nonsensical world of the Carroll's courtroom, the lizard juror writes notes with his finger from ink trickling down his face and the Red Queen shouts, "Sentence first – verdict afterwards" (Carroll & Gardner, 2000, p. 124). Alice is finally asked to leave because she is growing larger and larger, becoming too tall for the courtroom. Her increasing size suggests she is becoming too independent for the authorities in *Wonderland*. Feeling more daring and confident, Alice is no longer afraid of the autocratic Queen and wakes up.

I, too, found ways to grow independent of authority figures and find my own voice, including entering the world of psychology instead of the academic and scholarly field my father preferred for me. My choice was facilitated by my fascination with Alice's dream world, stimulating a life-long interest in dreams and the workings of the imagination and unconscious processes.

The character of Alice embodies what Phillips (2001) describes as the scientific Pragmatist and the artistic Dreamer. Carroll juxtaposed Alice's steady thoughtfulness – the Pragmatist, which comforted me – with a receptivity to strange happenings – the Dreamer, which gave me courage. This combination reflects how therapists are positioned: We are reliable and levelheaded, yet we have the audacity, as Alice did, to wander into the unconscious and interact with unpredictable and strange happenings.

My experience with Alice resonates with Arlene Richards and Lucille Spira (2015) *Myths of mighty women: Their application in psychoanalytic psychotherapy.* This volume details how female heroines in literature and myth can be used in psychotherapy to inspire women to give voice to their conflicts and gain emotional strength and assertiveness. For example, through a process of identification, patients can be inspired by a biblical character to take bold steps, as Miriam did as she danced and sang to lead her people and even dared to question her brother, Moses. Patients can also learn from literary characters what *not* to do, such as avoid the mourning process. We see the devastation this avoidance causes in the stifled life of Molly Bloom, the female character in James Joyce's *Ulysses.* At the point we meet Molly, she has been unable to mourn her son's death ten years earlier. The poignant story of Molly can revitalize the therapeutic dyad and help the patient gain the emotional strength to face loss.

Formal bibliotherapy uses works of fiction and nonfiction to address psychological problems and/or normal developmental issues. Numerous benefits have been reported (Afolayan, 1992; Hodges, 1995; Adler & Foster, 1997). Most authors, however, agree that the use of literature is an adjunct to psychotherapy, not a substitute for it (Holman, 1996). For an extensive discussion of the field of bibliotherapy, see John Pardeck (1998) and Dale Pehrsson and Paula McMillen (2005).

In a related vein, Fred Griffin (2016) argues that reading great literature can teach therapists how to listen analytically. Phillips (2001) argued similarly. He dedicates his book *Promises, Promises* to his literature teachers who, by teaching him to read, taught him how to listen. Griffin writes that our current emphasis on the importance of the intersubjective world has not been followed by enough education in how to listen in this new way. He proposes that psychoanalytic therapists read literature and gives specific suggestions for doing so. By entering the nuanced and highly textured worlds that writers such as Virginia Woolf create, the psychoanalytic therapist will learn to be more attuned to the patient's internal and relational worlds. This is a generative, imaginative form of reading and facilitates analytic sensibility.

"Psychoanalytic" live theater

Increasingly, drama therapy[11] is being used to direct attention to individual and collective trauma (Sajnani & Johnson, 2014). Drama therapy involves the use of theatrical techniques such as storytelling, projective play and performance to address psychological problems. Nisha Sajnani and David

Johnson identify the role of imagination as the healing factor in drama therapy. It invites patients to be receptive and to associate and create new ideas. Drama therapy is a two-step approach. As the dramatic story is performed, the trauma is conjured up. Then through the mechanisms of aesthetic distance, projective identification, playfulness, sharing, witnessing and discussion, the trauma is lessened and altered. It becomes more manageable.[12]

Expanding on the potential of therapeutic healing as a result of performance, Sally Bailey (2009, p. 376) writes, "Performing the story on a stage adds a formal sharing and witnessing aspect that provides another level of healing." The sense of a witnessing presence as the performance unfolds helps the viewer feel less alone. The use of projection allows audience members to experience in the characters some of their own dissociated states, helping them become aware of internal conflicts. The playful, make-believe aspect of the performance allows for greater self-acceptance. This all increases the capacity to recognize and bear the frustration and mental pain of trauma, necessary for growth (Fleming, 2008).

Intrigued by the potential of theater as a training, educational and therapeutic tool, I have written a number of plays, all of which deal with trauma. Art can provide "a 'witnessing' presence" (Rose, 1996, p. 1). In some ways similar to psychotherapy, it creates a sense of a responsive, holding other, helping the viewer experience a previously inaccessible aspect of self. I attempt to do this with my plays: to provide a holding environment for members of the audience to identify and work through trauma.

An example of self-revelatory theater (Emunah, 1994; Sharar, 2015), my first play, *The Meeting of My Dreams* (Domash, 2015), is loosely autobiographical and portrays the intergenerational transmission of conflict. Five generations of matriarchs from the same family meet (despite the fact that three are dead). At first, they inflict their conflicts on each other but then through the telling of dreams, begin to empathize with each other, and in some cases, forgive. During the "talk-back," members of the audience spontaneously identified and discussed their own experience of the intergenerational transmission of trauma. The members of the audience were very supportive of each other. The "talk back" became a safe, holding environment for the exploration and healing of family trauma for the audience and for myself as well.

The psychoanalytic relationship of Samuel Beckett and Wilfred Bion

An intriguing example of the healing possibilities of art is the therapeutic relationship of Samuel Beckett and Wilfred Bion and its aftermath. Beckett, age 28, became Bion's patient in early 1934 when both were at the beginning of their careers. Beckett would go on to become a highly esteemed playwright and novelist, winning the Nobel Prize for literature in 1969, and Bion, of course, an outstanding and profoundly influential theoretician-clinician.

At the point Beckett began analysis, he had begun a literary career but was struggling with a serious writing block and multiple emotional disturbances. He was tormented by, but could not separate from, his mother. He had a combination of long-standing interpersonal difficulties in close relationships and crippling somatic symptoms, including sleep disturbances and immobilizing fatigue (Simon, 1988). Beckett found the analytic experience difficult but did experience some relief, especially with his writing block. Later in his life he commented with gratitude that Bion had helped him through a very difficult period in his life (Beckett, 1985, personal communication with Bennett Simon).

After two years, Beckett broke off the analysis although the themes of his work with Bion – issues of meaning and human connection – preoccupied both men throughout their lives. Both Bennett Simon (1988) and Didier Anzieu (1989) examine Beckett's writing for allusions to his psychoanalysis and the working through of the negative transference. They conclude that Beckett continued to work on completing his abbreviated analysis with Bion through his writing, which served in part as a self-analysis and allowed him to continue to heal psychologically.

Referring to Beckett's novel *Murphy* (Beckett, 1994a), rewritten during his analysis with Bion and completed afterward in 1937, Simon (1988, p. 335) writes, "Treatment may not only have helped Beckett complete *Murphy*, but the writing of the book may have been in part a treatment." (See Bair, 1978; Ben-Zvi, 1986) In the novel, Murphy, an attendant in a psychiatric ward, and Mr. Endon, a nearly catatonic schizophrenic, play a game of chess. Simon (1998) suggests that the relationship between Murphy and Endon may reflect Beckett's feelings about his therapeutic work with Bion and that the interaction of these characters helped Beckett work through his conflicts.

Suffering a major reappearance of symptoms in 1943–1944, perhaps a psychotic episode, Beckett again appeared to benefit therapeutically from his writing. Beckett and his partner, Suzanne Déschevaux-Dumesnil, were hiding from the Nazis during World War II in southern France. During the years of occupation, Beckett worked in an underground resistance cell at great personal peril (Bair, 1978). During this time, Beckett (1994b) began writing the novel *Watt*, in part as an attempt at self-healing, and it seemed to be successful, just as writing *Murphy* helped him (Simon, 1988). He completed *Watt* in 1945.

In the novel, the character Watt, whose sanity is in question, confronts a puzzling lack of meaning in his interactions with others and with his surroundings. Working as a domestic servant, Watt is told by his employer, Mr. Knott to feed a dog when there is no dog. A door in the house is locked and then, mysteriously, unlocked. He is never able to connect to, or make sense of, Mr. Knott, at whose house "the true [is] true no longer, and the false not true yet" (Beckett, 1994b, p. 210). Finally, Watt enters a mental institution and has conversations with inmates where language gradually loses its meaning. The links between him and others are completely broken.

Addressing these issues may have helped Beckett work through fears of relatedness and connection, gaining necessary distance and a sense of mastery. Soon after completing *Watt*, Beckett enters one of his most productive periods, 1946–1950, when he wrote the novel trilogy *Molloy, Malone Dies* and *The Unnameable*[13] and the play *Waiting for Godot,*[14] the latter making him world famous.

Visual art and a new way of seeing

Frida Kahlo and self-analysis

Again, the question: can the artist do self-analysis? The renowned artist Frida Kahlo was traumatized at age 18 by a streetcar accident in which a metal bar entered her back and came out her vagina. As a result of the accident, she was unable to have children and in great physical pain throughout her life.[15] She began an explosive period of painting shortly after the accident, partly as an attempt to self-heal.

In her approximately 200 works, most were self-portraits. Transmuting her pain into remarkably original and dramatic imagery, Kahlo painted herself bleeding, weeping and cracked open. Her first task was the integration of her pre- and postaccident self. Concerning her shattered physical self or body ego, she was ingenious in physically recreating herself time and time again in self-portraits to help her maintain a cohesive, integrated sense of physical being. Because of its physicality, painting may be especially well suited to this. Another theme was her anguish concerning her inability to have children. There is an evolution of imagery in her paintings, which suggest a working through and ultimately a transformation of her feelings. In fact, her paintings seemed to become her productions, her children.

Commenting to an art critic[16] in 1944, Kahlo said that three concerns drove her to make art: "her vivid memory of her own blood flowing during her childhood accident; her thoughts about birth, death, and the 'conducting threads' of life; and her desire to be a mother" (Herrera, 1983, p. 319).

Able to do vital pieces of self-analysis with her art, Kahlo's work gave her an effective tool in her lifelong struggle between creation and destruction. At times, her painting functioned as a mirror transference would, restoring her sense of self. In moments of despair, the painting helped her bolster and maintain herself in the face of possible fragmentation. She was more successful using her art for psychological healing earlier in her life than later and more successful with narcissistic issues, that is, issues of the self, than with relational issues (Domash, 1990).

Her relational issues, especially with her mother, whom she felt to be rigid and distant, were not worked through in her art. These were mostly acted out repetitively in her stormy marriage to Diego Rivera and in her numerous affairs with both men and women (Domash, 1990). Sadly, her last years were filled with great physical and psychic pain, including an amputation of her right leg due to gangrene. She died in 1954 at age 47.

Art and the psychotherapist

Viewing art can help therapists expand their understanding of the psychotherapy process, by suggesting metaphorical connections. The Museum of Modern Art's 2016 exhibition *Edgar Degas: A Strange New Beauty* explored repetition and transformation, using monotypes. The artist draws in ink on a plate, which is sandwiched with a piece of paper and then run though a press. Typically, the artist sends a paper through only once, resulting in a single print. Each time there is a surprise, a "reveal."

However, using the same ink plate, Degas experimented and sent several papers through, sometimes adding color to these after-images. The images become more ghostly and surreal each time. In these ways he changed the image each time, playing with repetition and transformation, creating something that is the same yet different. This innovative process fascinated Degas. There is never a final product.

In psychotherapy, for both patient and therapist, some sessions are like the process of making a monotype, that is, the collection of thoughts, feelings and associations are pressed together and processed to create a new image or understanding. Many sessions have a "reveal," sometimes several. While patients change as a result of the therapeutic process, they also remain the same.

This relates to the practice of Embodied Imagination, in which the patient enters the landscape of her dream by embodying select images that eventually help transform her habitual way of seeing the world. Just like Degas dampened the paper to help it absorb the ink more easily, we help the patient become more receptive by inviting her into a hypnogogic state through a series of relaxation techniques. Then the therapist guides the patient to embody select images. These are eventually combined into a composite, which the patient mentally practices for weeks after the session. Embodying the dream images is like Degas' drawing on the plate while the continued practice of the composite is like the paper going through the press. This leads to change, and in many cases, transformation.

Degas was looking for techniques that would help him represent the new developments of his time. How do you portray a face illuminated by the new electric light? How do you portray a landscape seen from a moving train? How do you portray the smoke rising from stacks in the newly industrialized urban environment? The monotype helped him capture these moments. Like Degas in his day, therapists need to look for new approaches that will help their patients and themselves process the ever-changing internal and external landscape each faces on an on-going basis.

Another example of repetition with variation is Claude Monet's Haystacks, a series of approximately 30 works painted between 1890 and 1891. Monet portrayed the same haystack at various times of the day, through the seasons and in different types of weather. Each instance creates a mini-transformation. Monet teaches us to observe the nuances of change, seeing the same image at different times and in different moods, an invaluable skill for the therapist in her work.

Architecture and the creation of "therapeutic space"

Therapists usually think of transitional space as an *emotional* space, cocreated with their patients over the course of a treatment. This section, however, considers actual space as potential space, exploring how the physicality of architecture and design can transform. Because of its tendency to promote exploration and creative activity, architecture can create the facilitating environment needed to process emotion, regulate affect and reconceptualize narrative. An extension of psychoanalysis' recent appreciation of embodiment, architecture and design can contain as it reveals and help create novel personal and shared meanings in understanding the world.

In several articles, I examine the therapeutic effect of a major work of architecture, Daniel Libeskind's Jewish Museum in Berlin (Domash, 2014a, b). Long interested in the potential intersections of psychoanalysis and architecture, I had done a great deal of research on this structure, ultimately traveling to Berlin to experience its effect firsthand.

Although part of me was aware of harboring negative feelings toward Germany as a result of the Holocaust, I was nevertheless sideswiped by my response when my husband and I arrived in Berlin on a very cold and snowy evening in the middle of March 2013. Feeling surrounded by ghosts of the past and a history of horror, I was outraged by what I saw. This even included the cheerful, sickeningly sweet, pink aboveground water pipes laid throughout Berlin, which I viewed as a saccharine visual apology. Simultaneously, I began to feel self-hate, perhaps experiencing the feelings of the Jews of Berlin during WWII. Of course, the outrage I first experienced on this trip was not in response to the Germany of today but rather the Germany of many years ago.

The following day we made our way to the Jewish Museum. To stay with the metaphor, I entered the museum as a depressed, unhappy patient, and the effect of being there was like a powerful short-term dynamic therapy. We spent two full days in the museum: appreciating the permanent exhibit of 2,000 years of rich Jewish history in Germany, experiencing the voids of haunting empty spaces, doing research in the extensive learning center and, finally, listening to the eerie, atmospheric music installation based on Kafka's evocative aphorisms.

Approaching his design in a poetic, philosophical and psychological manner, Libeskind had to grapple with seemingly impossible questions and represent irreconcilable paradoxes. The Jews are an integral part of the history of Berlin and Germany yet were eliminated by the very culture to which they so heavily contributed. At this point in time, their presence in Germany is a mere fraction of what it once was. How to portray the Holocaust without becoming subsumed by it, or, even worse, reconciled? On an individual level, many of our patients face this same dilemma. They need to remember, to know on an emotional level, what happened in terms of their trauma; however, this is not to excuse or accept it. They need the strength to grasp it and, hopefully, recontextualize it.

Like a skilled therapist, Libeskind articulates these conundrums in a startling and arresting manner by conjuring a spatial experience of both fullness and emptiness. There is a zigzag design that is a powerful container for the narration of the nearly 2,000 years of Jewish life in Germany and the monumental contributions the Jews made to German culture. This visually beautiful narrative of fullness, richly symbolic with numerous interactive exhibits, served to tone down the experience of horror. Referencing back to psychotherapy, do therapists spend enough time on the positive introjections of their patients? On their positive accomplishments? It was from viewing the fullness of the German Jews' contributions that I gathered the strength to confront the ensuing emptiness more directly.

The narration of the fullness is contrasted with periodic voids representing the opposite, that of destruction and loss: expressions of the uncanny. They are set at intervals within a straight line running through the zigzag – symbolizing emptiness, cuts and disruptions. The spaces are black and empty; there are no exhibits in them. Frequently while standing inside in these spaces, one can look outside to an empty shaft of nothing, just air and light, representing absence – the destruction of the Jews. As Young (2000) states, the voids remind us of the dark abyss into which this culture once sank and from which it may never emerge.

While I was frightened, sad and tremendously angry as a result of confronting this huge loss, the feelings did not overwhelm me, due, in large part, to the thoughtfulness and artistry of the design. I was able to confront the horror of the Holocaust in the context of a safe haven, as in a good analytic session. Holding both of these states in mind provided integration and, in some way, helped me recontextualize my relationship to this history. I had the strength to bear it.

Thoughts for psychotherapy

Playfulness and interactivity

Despite the ubiquitous sense of trauma, the museum was playfully interactive, which also helped soften the sense of destruction, again reminding us of Winnicott's injunction that if the patient cannot play, the therapist must help him do so. In playing we are creative. We can reframe and recontextualize.

I was delighted to find an exhibit about a remarkable 17th-century woman named Glikl bas Juda Leib, mother of 14. She was equal to her husband in every way, and after he died, expanded his trading company and traveled widely. She also wrote her memoirs, comprising seven books, creating the oldest existing memoir written by a Jewish woman. The museum offers an opportunity for play by presenting a game that challenges the visitor to figure out what Glikl would take with her on her 17th-century business trips.

A large black glass box mounted to the wall offered another, more sinister experience. Designed by the artist Via Lewandowsky, it is an audio exhibit that recalls the "missing objects," the Jews. Although nothing can be seen in the black box, by moving one's body around in front of it, one can locate certain interactive spots, which then create sounds. We must search to "find" the missing objects, the lost souls.

The installation "Fallen Leaves" by the Israeli artist Menashe Kadishman is also noteworthy. He placed more than 10,000 metal faces in one of the museum's voids; the expressions on these faces tell the anguish of the victims. Visitors walk on the faces, and the movement of the metal creates eerie sounds, as if returning voice to the victims and allowing them to speak.

Repositioning the patient in "space"

Discussing how radical architecture reorients a person in physical space to have an entirely new experience in the world, Juliet MacCannell (2005) explores the work of the architect Emilio Ambasz, who wants to build "a house for the first man of a culture that has not yet arrived" (Wines, 2004, p. 86). He describes his work as the "pursuit of alternative models for a better future" (Wines, 2004, p. 108).

His buildings, such as The House of Spiritual Retreat (Casa Spiritual) in Spain, disorient and reorient perceptions in very creative ways. Creating a feeling of safety, steadiness and protection, the house is built entirely underground yet preserves the Spanish design of arranging rooms around a central courtyard. Light streams in from above. Above ground, one can climb a staircase up a high wall to see a glorious vista, inspiring a sense of future thinking. The whole experience is startlingly fresh and new.

According to MacCannell, the analyst, like the architect, can reposition the patient. She suggests viewing the patient's core unconscious fantasy from a spatial point of view. The analyst finds out where the patient is positioned in this "space" and attempts to reorient him, giving the patient greater flexibility and sense of possibility. This shift can help the patient gain perspective on his main issues and alter negative views about himself.

Similarly, Libeskind designed the spaces inside the museum to be "open narratives" (Young, 2000, p. 175), challenging preconceptions and providing the viewer with new, surprising ways to look at familiar material. Slanted walls and floors, black voids, oblique angles and stairs that lead nowhere all defamiliarize familiar ritual objects and historical chronologies, so the viewer can look at them as if for the first time.

Listening for surprise and state change

Exploring the architectural perspective in relation to psychoanalysis, Stephen Sonnenberg (2005) discusses the designer/artist/philosopher Cecil Balmond, who speaks of the "informal" environment, which promotes surprise and the potential for psychological state change in both the creator and user of a space. His structures encourage stepping out of a place fixed by conventional boundaries, which allows perceptions to mingle in spontaneous, vivid ways. As the architectural historian and critic Charles Jencks (2002) writes, Balmond pushes his structures in various ways so unexpected patterns emerge. Balmond wants the "sudden twist or turn" so "the edge of chance shows its face" (Balmond & Smith, 2002, p. 111). Sonnenberg writes that for Balmond, the building is a "vehicle opening up his mind to new, expansive ways of being, thinking, feeling, and designing" (Sonnenberg, 2005, p. 47).

Sonnenberg advocates that psychoanalysis could become even more compatible with the goals of the "informal." The analyst can listen to the patient in a manner that welcomes the possibility of new, surprising ideas and changes in psychological state that may facilitate sudden growth in the patient. We have spoken of the usual slow, gradual process in psychotherapy. Yet there can also be times of rapid, unexpected growth.

Our visit comes to an end

Art is transformative. Art allows for greater recognition and acceptance of dissociated states. Serving as a witnessing presence, art can reduce loneliness and restore the sense of an empathic internal other, so often lost in trauma. Art can provide therapeutic distance, allowing the patient to gain perspective. Art helps integrate split aspects of the self as well as process emotion and facilitate mourning, as in the case of Frida Kahlo.

The arts remind the therapeutic dyad of the importance of thoughtfulness, of playfulness and interactivity, of listening for surprise, and of focusing on positive developments as well as trauma. This allows the patient to reflect, tolerate ambiguity, reorient himself within his narrative and finally, allow change. Art, as well as psychotherapy, can inspire patients to create what is longed for but previously thought impossible.

Notes

1 Parts of this chapter appeared in an earlier version in Domash, (2014a) and Domash (2014b) and are gratefully reprinted with permission from Taylor & Francis.

2 In the paranoid schizoid stage, persecutory anxiety is prominent; the main defenses are splitting and projection. The Other is related to as a fragmented part-object that satisfies immediate needs, such as the infant viewing the mother mainly as a breast. In the depressive position, considered by Klein to be a movement beyond the paranoid schizoid, the ability to integrate increases and the

capacity for concern develops. The Other is now related to as a whole person, and the capacity to feel loss, guilt and dependence emerges (Klein, 1946, 1948; Steiner, 1979). The depressive position has recently been renamed the reparative position by psychoanalyst Donald Carveth (2018).

3 Akhtar (2000, p. 229) describes mental pain as consisting of "... a wordless sense of self-rupture, longing and psychic helplessness that is vague and difficult to convey to others." Freud used the term *Seelenschmerz*, literally meaning soul-pain, to discuss this concept. Freud likened mental pain to the helplessness and longing in the cries of a baby for his mother (Freud, 1926).

4 Yeats, W.B. (2002). The Lake Isle of Innisfree. In R.J. Finneran (Ed.), *The Yeats reader: A portable compendium of poetry, drama, and prose* (pp. 13–14). New York: Scribner.

5 Hopkins, G.M. (2009). My Own Heart. In C. Phillips (Ed.), *Gerard Manley Hopkins: The major works* (p. 170). New York: Oxford University Press.

6 Dickinson, E. (1976). Wild nights! Wild nights! In T.H. Johnson (Ed.), *The collected poems of Emily Dickinson* (p. 114). New York: Little, Brown.

7 Williams, W.C. (1991). The Red Wheelbarrow. In A.W. Litz & C. MacGowan (Eds.), *The collected poems of William Carlos Williams: Volume 1: 1909–1939* (p. 224). New York: New Directions.

8 Cummings, E.E. (1994). I thank You God for most this amazing. In R.S. Kennedy (Ed.), *Selected Poems* (p. 167). New York: Norton.

9 Oliver, M.(Ed.) (2017). The Journey. In *Devotions: The selected poems of Mary Oliver* (pp. 349–350). New York: Penguin.

10 Fleischman, P. (text) & Beddows, E. (illustrations). (1988). Chrysalis Diary. In *Joyful noise: Poems for two voices* (pp. 39–44). New York: Harper and Row.

11 Drama therapy can take a number of forms: (1) playback theater: an audience member tells a moment from his or her life, choses the actors to play the roles and then watches the performance (Rowe, 2007; Salas, 2013); (2) self-revelatory performance: a performer originates a theatre piece drawn from current problematic life issues and produces a work that is performed (Emunah, 2015); (3) psychodrama: uses guided drama and role playing to process problems in a group setting (Moreno, 1964; Blatner, 2000) and is as effective or more effective than traditional group psychotherapy (Kipper & Ritchie, 2003); and (4) therapeutic theater: usually performed by a group of people frequently seen as marginalized who share concerns. Performances are not necessarily based on real life and can provide a sense of mastery (Emunah, 1994; Sajnani, 2013).

12 For more information on drama therapy, consult the website of the North American Drama Therapy Association (NADTA), http://www.nadta.org There is a vast literature on drama therapy (Irwin, 1982; Emunah & Johnson, 1983; Landy, 1983, 1996, 2003; Cattanach, 1993, 2008; Jennings, 1994; Seligman, 1995; Emunah, 1997; Herman, 1997; James & Johnson, 1997; Glass, 2006; Stahler, 2006/2007; Bloch, 2007; Jones, 2007, 2010; Bailey, 2009; Sajnani, 2010; Butler, 2012; Chapman, 2014; Emunah et al., 2014 and others).

13 Beckett, S. (2009). L. Lingren (Ed.), *Three novels: Molloy, Malone dies, The unnamable.* New York: Grove Press.

14 Beckett, S. (2011). *Waiting for Godot: A tragicomedy in two acts*. New York: Grove Press.

15 Biographical information concerning Frida Kahlo's life is taken from the excellent work by Hayden Herrera (1983).

16 Identified only as A.F. in "Frida Kahlo y Melancholia de la Sangre" ("Frida Kahlo and the Melancholy of Blood") in the magazine *Rueca*, Mexico City, 1944, 10:80.

References

Adler, E.S. & Foster, P. (1997). A literature-based approach to teaching values to adolescents: Does it work? *Adolescence*, 32(126):275–287.Afolayan, J.A. (1992). Documentary perspective of bibliography in education. *Reading Horizons*, 33(2):137–148.

Akhtar, S. (2000). Mental pain and the cultural ointment of poetry. *International Journal of Psycho-Analysis*, 81(2):229–243.

Anzieu, D. (1989). Beckett and Bion. *International Review of Psycho-Analysis*, 16:163–169.

Arieti, S. (1976). *Creativity: The magic synthesis*. New York: Basic Books.

Bailey, S. (2009). Performance in drama therapy. In D.R. Johnson & R. Emunah (Eds.), *Current approaches in drama therapy*, Second edition (pp. 375–389). Springfield: Charles C Thomas Publisher.

Bair, D. (1978). *Samuel Beckett: A biography*. New York: Harcourt Brace Jovanovich.

Balmond, C. & Smith, J. (2002). *Informal*. Munich: Prestel Verlag.

Beckett, S. (1985). Personal communication with Bennett Simon.

Beckett, S. (1994a). *Murphy*. New York: Grove Press.

Beckett, S. (1994b). *Watt*. New York: Grove Press.

Ben-Zvi, L. (1986). *Samuel Beckett*. Boston, MA: Twayne Publishing.

Blatner, A. (2000). *Foundation of psychodrama*. New York: Springer.

Bloch, S. (2007). Reflections: A teen issues improv troupe. In A. Blatner & D.J. Wiener (Eds.), *Interactive and improvisational drama: Varieties of applied theatre and performance* (pp. 56–65). New York: iUniverse, Inc.

Bollas, C. (1978). The aesthetic moment and the search for transformation. *Annual of Psychoanalysis*, 6:385–394.

Bollas, C. (2011a). Creativity and psychoanalysis. In *The Christopher Bollas reader* (pp. 194–206). New York: Routledge.

Bollas, C. (Ed.) (2011b). The transformational object. In *The Christopher Bollas reader* (pp. 1–12). New York: Routledge.

Breton, A. (1969). *Manifestoes of surrealism*. Ann Arbor: University of Michigan Press.

Butler, J.D. (2012). Playing with madness: Developmental transformations and the treatment of schizophrenia. *The Arts in Psychotherapy*, 39(2):87–94.

Carroll, L. (2000). J. Gardner (Introduction and notes), *The annotated Alice: The definitive edition*. Original illustrations by J. Tenniel. New York: Norton.

Carveth, D. (2018). *Psychoanalytic thinking: A dialectical critique of contemporary theory and practice*. New York: Routledge.

Cattanach, A. (1993). The developmental model of dramatherapy. In S. Jennings, A. Cattanach, S. Mitchell, A. Chesner & B. Meldrum (Eds.), *The handbook of dramatherapy* (pp. 28–40). New York: Routledge.

Cattanach, A. (2008). Working creatively with children and their families after trauma: The restoried life. In C.A. Malchiodi (Ed.), *Creative interventions with traumatized children* (pp. 211–224). New York: Guilford Press.

Chapman, E.J. (2014). Using dramatic reality to reduce depressive symptoms: A qualitative study. *The Arts in Psychotherapy*, 41(2): 137–144.

Dali, S. (2007). *Diary of a genius*. Chicago, IL: Solar Books.

Domash, L. (November 9, 1990). Working with trauma: The self-analysis of Frida Kahlo. Colloquium, The New York University Postdoctoral Program of Psychotherapy and Psychoanalysis, New York, NY.
Domash, L. (2014a). Creating "therapeutic" space: How architecture and design can inform psychoanalysis. *Psychoanalytic Perspectives*, 11: 94–111.
Domash, L. (2014b). Intergenerational dreaming: Response to Gerald and Sperber. *Psychoanalytic Perspectives*, 11:133–137.
Domash, L. (2015). The meeting of my dreams (theatrical presentation). Performances: April 26, 2015, 35th Annual Spring Meeting of the Division of Psychoanalysis (39) of the American Psychological Association, *Life in Psychoanalysis in Life*; July 19, 2015, Society for Exploration of Psychoanalytic Therapies and Theology, Allentown, PA.
Dubrasky, D., Sorensen, S., Donovan, A. & Corser, G. (2019). "Discovering inner strengths": A co-facilitative poetry therapy curriculum for groups. *Journal of Poetry Therapy*, 32(1):1–10.
Emunah, R. (1994). *Acting for real: Drama therapy process, technique, and performance.* New York: Brunner/Mazel.
Emunah, R. (1997). Drama therapy and psychodrama: An integrated model. *International Journal of Action Methods: Psychodrama, Skill Training, and Role Playing*, 50(3):108–134.
Emunah, R. (2015). Self-revelatory performance: A form of drama therapy and theatre. *Drama Therapy Review*, 1(1): 71–85.
Emunah, R. & Johnson, D.R. (1983). The impact of theatrical performance on the self-images of psychiatric patients. *The Arts in Psychotherapy*, 10: 233–239.
Emunah, R., Raucher, G. & Ramirez-Hernandex, A. (2014). Self-revelatory performance in mitigating the impact of trauma. In N. Sajnani & D.R. Johnson (Eds.), *Trauma-informed drama therapy: Transforming clinics, classrooms, and communities* (pp. 93–121). Springfield, IL: Charles C. Thomas Publisher.
Fleming, M. (2008). On mental pain: From Freud to Bion. *International Journal of Psycho-Analysis*, 17(1): 27–36.
Freud, S. (1926). Inhibitions, symptoms and anxiety. *Standard Edition*, 20:77–175.
Glass, J. (2006). Working toward aesthetic distance: Drama therapy for adult victims of trauma. In L. Carey (Ed.), *Expressive and creative arts methods for trauma survivors* (pp. 57–71). London: Jessica Kingsley Publishers.
Glover, N. (2009). *Psychoanalytic aesthetics: An introduction to the British School.* London: Karnac.
Griffin, F.L. (2016). *Creative listening and the psychoanalytic process: Sensibility, engagement, envisioning.* New York: Routledge.
Herman, L. (1997). Good enough fairy tales for resolving sexual abuse trauma. *The Arts in Psychotherapy*, 24(5):439–445.
Herrera, H. (1983). *Frida: A biography of Frida Kahlo.* New York: Harper and Row.
Heines, S. (2011). State of poetry therapy research. *The Arts in Psychotherapy*, 38:1–8.
Hodges, J. (1995). *Conflict resolution for the young child.* (ERIC document Reproduction Service ED 394 624).
Holman, W.D. (1996). The power of poetry: Validating ethnic identity through a bibliotherapeutic intervention with a Puerto Rican adolescent. *Child and Adolescent Social Work Journal*, 13(5):371–383.
Irwin, E.C. (1982). Enlarging the psychodynamic picture through dramatic play techniques. In K. O'Laughlin & E. Nickerson (Eds.), *Helping through action:*

Readings on action-oriented therapies (pp. 53–59). Amherst, MA: Human Resource Development Press.
James, M. & Johnson, D.R. (1997). Drama therapy in the treatment of combat-related posttraumatic stress disorder. *The Arts in Psychotherapy*, 23(5):383–395.
Jencks, C. (2002). Preface: Changing architecture. In C. Balmond & J. Smith (Eds.), *Informal* (pp. 5–8). Munich: Prestel Verlag.
Jennings, S. (1994). What is dramatherapy? Interviews with pioneers and practitioners. In S. Jennings, A. Cattanach, S. Mitchell, A. Chesner & B. Meldrum (Eds.), *The handbook of dramatherapy* (pp. 166–186). New York: Routledge.
Jones, P. (2007). *Drama as therapy volume 1: Theory, practice and research*. New York: Routledge.
Jones, P. (2010). *Drama as therapy volume 2: Clinical work and research into practice*. New York: Routledge.
Klein, M. (1946). Notes on some schizoid mechanisms. *International Journal of Psycho-Analysis*, 27:99–110.
Klein, M. (1948). *Contributions to psycho-analysis 1921–1945*. London: Hogarth Press.
Kipper, D.A. & Ritchie, T.D. (2003). The effectiveness of psychodramatic techniques: A meta-analysis. *Group Dynamics Theory Research and Practice*, 7(1): 13–25.
Landy, R.J. (1983). The use of distancing in drama therapy. *The Arts in Psychotherapy*, 10(3):175–185.
Landy, R.J. (1996). *Essays in drama therapy: The double life*. Philadelphia, PA: Jessica Kingsley Publishers.
Landy, R.J. (2003). Drama therapy with adults. In C.E. Schaefer (Ed.), *Play therapy with adults* (pp. 15–33). New York: Wiley.
Laub, D. & Podell, D. (1995). Art and trauma. *International Journal of Psycho-analysis*, 76:991–1005.
Lispector, C. (2012). *Aqua viva*. New York: New Directions.
Longley, M. (November 3, 2016). Interview with Krista Tippet. *On Being*.
MacCannell, J.F. (2005). FreudSpace architecture in psychoanalysis. *Annual of Psychoanalysis*, 33:93–107.
Modell, A. (2006). *Imagination and the meaningful brain*. Cambridge, MA: MIT Press.
Moreno, J.L. (1964). *Psychodrama: Vol. 1*. Beacon, NY: Beacon.
O'Conner, S.M., Nikoletti, L.J., Kristjanson, R. & Wilcock, B. (2003). Writing therapy for the bereaved: Evaluation of an intervention. *Journal of Palliative Medicine*, 6(2):195–204.
Ogden, T.H. (1994). The analytic third: Working with intersubjective clinical facts. *International Journal of Psycho-Analysis*, 75:3–19.
Ogden, T.H. (1998). A question of voice in poetry and psychoanalysis. *Psychoanalytic Quarterly*, 67(3):426–448.
Pardeck, J.T. (1998). *Using books in clinical social work practice: A guide to bibliotherapy*. New York: Haworth.
Pehrsson, D. & McMillen, P.S. (2005). A bibliotherapy evaluation tool: Grounding counselors in the therapeutic use of literature. *The Arts in Psychotherapy*, 32(1):47–59.
Pennebaker, J.W., Kiecolt-Glaser, J. & Glase, R. (1988). Disclosure of traumas and immune function: Health implication for psychotherapy. *Journal of Consulting and Clinical Psychology*, 56: 239–245.

Phillips, A. (2001). *Promises, promises: Essays on psychoanalysis and literature*. New York: Basic Books.

Proulx, T. & Heine, S.J. (2009). Connections from Kafka: Exposure to meaning threats improves implicit learning of an artificial grammar. *Psychological Science*, 20(9):1125–1131.

Pynchon, P. (1998). *Slow learner: Early stories*. New York: Little Brown.

Rafferty, C. (August 2, 2015). Book review of *The Complete Stories*. *New York Times*, Sunday Book Review.

Richards, A.K. & Spira, L. (2015). *Myths of mighty women: Their application in psychoanalytic psychotherapy*. London: Karnac.

Rose, G.J. (1996). *Necessary illusion: Art as witness*. New York: International Universities Press.

Rowe, N. (2007). *Playing the other: Dramatizing personal narratives in playback theater*. London: Jessica Kingsley.

Sajnani, N. (2010). Mind the gap. Facilitating transformative witnessing amongst audiences. In P. Jones (Ed.), *Drama as therapy, Volume 2: Clinical work and research into practice* (pp. 189–207). London: Routledge.

Sajnani, N. (2013). The body politic: The relevance of an intersectional framework for therapeutic performance research in drama therapy. *The Arts in Psychotherapy*, 40(3):382–385.

Sajnani, N. & Johnson, D.R. (2014). *Trauma-informed drama therapy: Transforming clinics, classrooms, and communities*. Springfield: Charles C. Thomas.

Salas, J. (2013). *Improvising real life: A personal story in playback theatre*. New Paltz: Tusilata.

Seligman, Z. (1995). Trauma and drama: A lesson from the concentration camp. *The Arts in Psychotherapy*, 22(2):119–132.

Sharar, J. (February 10, 2015). Drama therapy meets psychoanalysis. *Linkedin*. https://www.linkedin.com/pulse/drama-therapy-meets-psychoanalysis-jarred-sharar

Simon, B. (1988). The imaginary twins: The case of Beckett and Bion. *International Review of Psychoanalysis*, 15:331–352.

Sonnenberg, S.M. (2005). What can psychoanalysis learn from an enhanced awareness of architecture and design? *Annual of Psychoanalysis*, 33:39–56.

Stahler, W. (2006/2007). Prayerformance: A drama therapy approach with female prisoners recovering from addiction. *Journal of Creativity in Mental Health*, 2(1):3–12.

Steiner, J. (1979). The border between the paranoid-schizoid and the depressive positions in the borderline patient. *British Journal of Medical Psychology*, 52:385–391.

Tegner, I., Fox, J., Philipp, R. & Thorne, P. (2009). Evaluating the use of poetry to improve well-being and emotional resilience in cancer patients. *Journal of Poetry Therapy*, 22(9):121–131.

Young, J. (2000). *At memory's edge: After-Images of the holocaust in contemporary art and literature*, New Haven, CT: Yale University Press.

Wallach, M. (2003). In search of the poetic analyst. *Journal of the American Academy of Psychoanalysis*, 31:397–409.

Wines, J. (2004). Emilio Ambasz: Soft and hard. In M. Sorkin (Ed.), *Analyzing Ambasz* (pp. 86–108). New York: Monacelli Press.

Winnicott, D.W. (1971). *Playing and reality.* London: Tavistock.
Woolf, V. (1971). Lewis Carroll. In R. Phillips (Ed.), *Aspects of Alice: Lewis Carroll's dreamchild as seen through the critics' looking-glasses, 1865–1971* (pp. 47–49). New York: Vanguard.
Zelnick, L. (2014). Narrative surprise: Relational psychoanalytic process and biblical text. *DIVISION/Review*, 9:33.

Chapter 9

Desire's arousal

In *Wonderland*, Alice inspires us to consider the importance of dreams, the potential of language and the value of tolerating the unknown. Alice shows us how fairy tales and make-believe can be very real and how not to interpret life too literally. You and I have wandered down into this unconscious dreamworld and, hopefully, both changed as a result. We begin and end in *Wonderland*.

Yet there is no need to say goodbye. This is only the beginning of desire's arousal: the desire to know *more* and *less* at the same time, to enter the world of dreams, to play with language, to experience surprise, to contain and reveal, to discover your voice, and to converse with other disciplines. As you continue the practice of psychotherapy, I invite you return to this volume for inspiration and contemplation. Clinicians are entrusted with the souls of their patients and need nourishment to care for them.

Surprise

The crucial importance of welcoming surprise, and even generating environments in which both patient and analyst can experience the unexpected, has been emphasized by many psychoanalytic writers (Reik, 1936; Stern, 1990; Bromberg, 2000; Domash, 2009, 2010 among others). From time to time, either side of the therapeutic dyad can find herself in what Zelnick (2014, p. 33) terms a "relational double take," a dramatic surprise about the other or oneself. I experienced this with Alice. My dreamy state as I descended down the rabbit hole opened me up to *Wonderland's* multiple surprises – Alice's bizarre size changes, the Red Queen's imperious shouts, the Duchess' cruelty, the Cheshire's cat surreal grin and the baby who becomes a pig. I remember being very drawn in as each nonsensical surprise served to broaden my narrow view and see new possibilities. Surprise, even absurdity, can facilitate learning.

Containment

Wonderland creates a container for fragments of feelings states that may not have yet come to consciousness. Surprise requires containment. In her topsy-turvy, unpredictable world, Alice helped me articulate hopes for a more interesting life. I agreed with her that "It seemed quite dull and stupid for life to go on in the common way" (Carroll, 2000, p. 19). She had begun to think, "that very few things indeed were really impossible" (Carroll, 2000, p. 16). I believed her that something interesting was bound to happen.

Similarly, the therapeutic experience serves a containment function, an analytic process first described by Bion (1962) in which the analyst is able to hold the unmanageable, inchoate projections of the patient and then reflect them back to her. This bidirectional flow allows the patient to tolerate the psychoanalytic experience, and thoughts can be born.

The patient frequently comes to treatment encased in dysphoric, dissociated space with little sense of containment. We begin by containing the patient in the sacred space of our office. The act of "havdalah,"[1] the Hebrew word for separation, is central. Entering the psychotherapy office is a separation from the outside world and becomes a home for the unconscious – Jung's concept of temenos[2] – where one's innermost thoughts and feelings are welcome. Functioning in both known and unknown space, the therapist coaxes the patient into dream space while providing regulation and insight. The therapist translates the patient's terror space into manageable space for him to ponder.

You, as the reader of this volume, also exist in "book-space" with me, in an ever-deepening appreciation of unconscious processes at work. I aim to stimulate your desire to know as much as you can and, at the same time, be comfortable not knowing, a blank slate upon which the patient can write his story.

Finding one's voice

Alice's voice is curious and open yet also reasonable and thoughtful. Changing over the course of the novel, her voice is at first timid, then gradually more daring and confident. This is clearly seen at the end when she speaks out about the absurdity of the trial, and she is no longer afraid of the Red Queen. "Who cares for you," Alice says to the Red Queen, "You're nothing but a pack of cards!" (Carroll, 2000, p. 124). This development inspired me as a young reader.

Alice encouraged me to be "curiouser and curiouser!" (Carroll, 2000, p. 20), to think and question yet welcome all this dream strangeness. Looking back, what appealed to me most was the juxtaposition of Alice's steady thoughtfulness (which comforted me) with her openness to the strange happenings (which gave me courage). This is how therapists are positioned: reliable and levelheaded yet with the audacity to wander into the unconscious and interact with unpredictable and surprise happenings.

I encourage the clinician to travel to her unconscious dream world, gather her unique viewpoint, her signature style and her poetic vision. She must find her words and help the patient find his. This is crucial to the development of the patient's sense of self, his relation to others and his ability to find passion in love and work. Capturing my voice was my struggle in writing this book. (Remember my dream horse in Chapter 6 covered with hay, working to break free?)

Mentors help, as creativity is in part a relational process. The mentor can inspire and guide and reduce anxiety. Clinicians are mentors for their patients. The therapist has an intuitive sense of the use of psychic heat to help the patient develop – when to get louder and hotter and when to be softer and cooler.

Inspiration

It is important for the clinician to find nourishing inspiration for himself and his patient. Turning to the poets, when e.e. cummings thanks God for the beauty of the trees and sky,[3] he is grateful for the everyday and sees it illuminated. When William Carlos Williams gazes at a red wheelbarrow after a rain,[4] who does not feel his wonder?

Many patients come to psychotherapy feeling alienated and anxious, even shattered and need inspiration and emotional nourishment to develop trust and faith in the process. Faith ushers us into transitional space and activates the placebo effect. If one has faith in a treatment, it frequently will work. The activation of faith poises the patient to work on lessening dissociation and/or repression, so he or she can become more integrated and complete.

The dyad can find faith and nourishment in the arts. The patient writing about a traumatic event may help her contain anxiety, gain perspective and feel less lonely. Art provides a witnessing presence, an empathic other, so frequently lost in trauma. Writing a poem about a patient may help the clinician see the patient from the inside out. As she searches to find image words to express her grasp of the patient, she gains increased empathy. The aesthetic distance may also help her reflect on a potential enactment.

The lack that sparks desire

The serpent (possibly sent by God) seduced Eve into wanting more. Alice coaxed me into contemplating strangeness. Clinicians work to activate desire in the patient to seek and find what is missing. We offer the patient an inviting atmosphere, a space apart, to learn about what he may need and how he might engage with the world.

Many patients come to treatment with an agitated and/or numb sense that something is lacking. Wallace Stevens famously wrote that desire begins in not having.[5] If and when the patient's feeling of lack sparks desire, this can ignite the treatment. However, the feeling of desire can be frightening, as the object of desire has power. Many patients chose not to interact in meaningful ways in the world for fear of this loss of power. The clinician works with the patient to tolerate and, perhaps, even embrace desire.

The therapist also desires to know the patient. This is paradoxical as there is a desire not to know at the same time. The therapist keeps desire alive by knowing there is always more to know. George Steiner (1989) considers that while art aims to attenuate a sense of strangeness (in therapy terms, "to know"), it also works to make strangeness in certain respects stranger ("to not know"). Therapists work to help the patient feel less alien and more integrated yet also work to create a strangeness to keep desire alive for new insights to be found. There are always familiarities and mysteries in the narrative of the patient.

The potter and his clay

The clinician guides the way yet the patient has control as well. This is similar to the interactions between the artist and his material and in biblical scholar Zornberg's reflections, between God and man (Zornberg, 1995). As is described in the Book of Jeremiah, while the potter makes the clay pot (and in some sense has control), the pot also tells the potter what it wants to be. Zornberg (1995) writes that even God sacrifices some of his sovereignty when he makes man in his image. God is willing to contract to create space for the world because he desires to be known by man. However, now man has free will and may not always do God's bidding.

Adam, too, sacrifices some of his power when Eve is created. Yet Adam desires a partner as without one, life might be static and unchanging. Adam and Eve get to live face-to-face with each other – uniting and separating according to their will. They have the benefits of loving involvement but the risks of vulnerability.

Both patient and therapist give up aspects of their "freedom." While the patient may feel understood and validated, and in that sense "free," he is also required to be vulnerable, accept challenge and even more difficult, attempt change. He is face-to-face with the therapist, intertwined in union and separateness. There are risks and freedoms for the therapist as well. She is free to make observations and interpretations yet is also humbled by the expressions and proclivities of the patient. Patient and therapist dance together, with the therapist leading but always cognizant if she and the patient are in step.

The hum in the ear

In relation to biblical texts, Zornberg describes the interpretative act as a creative act, requiring vigorous imaginative effort. Such is also the case with psychotherapy. This process begins with the therapist's "sense" of what is happening – with the "hum in the ears" (Zornberg, 1995, p. xix), the feeling in the gut – as she tries to catch something from an unknown source and put it into words.

Zornberg uses the phrase "hum in the ears" in reference to Nadezhda Mandelstam's account of how her husband, Osip Mandelstam, the esteemed Russian poet and activist, would begin a new poem. He would hear a musical phrase repeatedly ring in his ears, at first formless but then begin to take shape. He appeared to feel as if he were receiving something from an unknown source, which slowly shaped itself into words.

The clinician's intuition is similar. Some feelings start to swirl around, not clear, maybe foolish, but they linger and coalesce. At times, they too seem to be coming not from within but from elsewhere, as I describe in Chapter 3. The clinician considers them and waits to see if further work reveals them to be accurate. I frequently use the initial telephone call and first few sessions to form a hypothesis about the patient, which I test out in subsequent sessions.

Bollas (2017) writes about the unthought known, hints of which are in the free associations of the patient, in fragments of the transference and countertransference and in the resonance or lack thereof between patient and analyst. Who is the analyst to the patient and vice versa? Grappling with the unthought known creates desire in the dyad for meaning.

Bollas states that transference may be more than what we originally thought, that is, not only a rerepresentation of what has already been experienced but also elements of psychic life that have not yet been thought and therefore new for the patient. Much of this information is beneath the level of awareness yet known unconsciously, hence the unthought known. This includes the parts of the patient's true self which have not yet been lived, perhaps repressed or dissociated. With time, the clinician facilitates these parts coming to consciousness. In this instance, the analyst is a transformational object (Bollas, 1979), much as original caretakers are, as they help facilitate the true self into being.

The spiritual imagination

In psychotherapy, as in *Wonderland*, the ordinary can transmute into the extraordinary. Implicit feelings of spirituality emerge in our work as patient and therapist interact in potential space. In this realm, the dyad has a sense of connection that goes beyond the ordinary. Barriers can come down and self-states become more integrated. This developing spiritual imagination allows the patient to experiment with rearranging long established dysfunctional patterns and create a new emotional landscape.

When therapists enter this space with patients, they are activating right brain functioning in the context of an attachment relationship, helping the patient self-regulate and gain access to imagistic thinking and visual metaphor. As Marks-Tarlow (2012, p. 162) writes, "Allan Schore views imagery, symbolic thought, and the visual imagination as the apex of 'high right' functioning." If entrance into this space is successful, the dyad can see beyond the literal. They are open to surprise. They can be amazed.

The Kabbalah teaches that God represents deep structure while man represents surface – in our terms, latent/manifest, implicit/explicit, unconscious/conscious (Starr, 2008). Students of Kabbalah work to connect with this deeper structure by knowing themselves fully. This develops the divine spark or godliness within (the "gold" of the alchemists), which is at first hidden from consciousness. Therapists work to help the patient find his whole (holy) self. In this sense, therapists have a sacred responsibility in the therapeutic relationship.

The writing of this book has been a spiritual journey for me. I have been engrossed in a state of flow (Csikszentmihalyi, 1996), living in the transitional realm, as I write, struggle, despair, clarify and overcome. I am always thinking of how to better connect and communicate with you, my reader, as well as how much to reveal. I have striven to achieve the best balance, so my personal discussions can help you move toward your own vision with flair and resourcefulness.

The relational/resonant imagination

The relational/resonant imagination allows the therapist to build the therapeutic relationship and foster faith and trust. Sensing what is hidden in the spaces between the words, the therapist grasps the nonverbal communication of the patient: the change in tone of voice, the side-glance, the shift in the seat, the odd question. This involves body-to-body communication, as Knoblauch (2005) describes when he turns his attention to the shifts of movement and sound in his patient's body as they resonate with his own.

Just as a sensitive biblical reader does, the clinician "reads" the patient and encourages him to yield up his meanings. Zornberg's desire is "to loosen the fixities, the ossifications of preconceived readings" (Zornberg, 1995, p. xii) of the bible. Zornberg therefore works to find instability within stability and disorder within order, as a therapist might with a patient who has difficulty veering from his fixed habitual view of the world. For Zornberg, the Torah text can only really be known by the strenuous imaginative thinking of the biblical reader. Therapists, too, need a strenuous relational imagination to know the patient.

"Aha" moments spring from the relational unconscious, when something in the therapist's unconscious suddenly shifts and gives him the freedom to respond to the patient with new insight. In these instances, the therapist receives the unconscious, nonverbal communication of the patient, processes it out of awareness, and suddenly, without previous conscious thought, reformulates her understanding in a novel and clear way.

Thoughts may pass between you and your patient, as if you are reading each other's minds. As Marks-Tarlow (2012) writes, we are intertwined with our patient beneath the level of awareness. There are also clinical reports of uncanny unconscious communication at a distance, when a patient or therapist becomes aware of something about the other when not in each other's presence.

While some of these phenomena are seemingly telepathic and not well understood, they can be extremely therapeutic, helping both sides of the dyad break free from the familiar and welcome the unexpected. They also give us clues to less understood aspects of therapeutic communication and action, including projective identification, therapeutic intuition, transference/countertransference enactments and intersubjectivity.

In addition to intuiting the patient and sensing his unconscious, the therapist must communicate relevant information back to the patient in a manner that can be accepted and processed. Warren Poland (1975) discusses the importance of psychoanalytic tact, which refers to *how* a statement is made, based on an empathic connection to the patient. It also encompasses silences and nonverbal communication. Ideally, therapists sense the language and intensity needed for a particular moment, ranging from a deeply soothing empathic comment to the implicit aggression in an interpretation.

As Poland writes, we may be in the position of telling the patient something he does not want to hear, especially if it means giving up narcissistic gratification. An underlying experience of warm acceptance helps the patient tolerate the shame of exposing vulnerabilities to explore new insights. Tact allows the therapist/analyst to reveal disquieting qualities about the patient while at the same time protect the patient's self-esteem. This encourages self-reflection.

Clinicians are aware of countertransference disturbances of tact. Errors of judgment are made when unresolved anger or narcissism cause either an inhibition in the clinician to guard against his own sadism or a breakthrough of anger in overt verbal aggression. The same can be said for sexuality. If tact fails in this regard, the therapist may become seductive or, as a defense, distant and cold. This is not to say that tact is a panacea. It may be difficult to reach some patients no matter how tactful the therapist. Further, the therapist may not have the skill or language for a particular patient.

Dreamwork

Patients frequently enter treatment trapped in dysfunctional patterns created by early unconscious memories. Our task is to help them learn new patterns. Much like Alice, they have to tolerate the anxiety of changing and growing. Alice changes size 12 times. This suggests she has to learn to shift perspectives and experience unusual viewpoints, as in Embodied Imagination dreamwork, to mature and grow up.

Whether solving an emotional, aesthetic or scientific problem, dreamwork is one key to accessing unconscious memories and using them in new ways. Embodied Imagination encourages deep entrance into dream images, especially ones that are alien to the dreamer, and creates new networks and patterns to replace old dysfunctional ones. It facilitates creative projects by breaking the habitual frame of the dreamer and opening up pathways heretofore not experienced.

Alice's Adventures in Wonderland provides an opportunity to live in the unconscious, that is, to experience a very long dream and learn from it. Bosnak views all the parts of the dream not as aspects of the self but as individual subjectivities from which one can learn. In this way, *Wonderland* offered multiple learning opportunities to this seven- or eight-year-old who was too literal and not sure how to think for herself.

Dreams and poetry are so close. The vivid imagery, the intensity, the unusual combinations, the surreal quality and the directness we find in dreams can be thought of as visual poetry. As the writer Jean Paul Richter said, "Dreams are an involuntary form of poetry" (as quoted in Darwin, 1879/2004, p. 95). Psychotherapy and poetry employ imaginative leaping, offer startling or unexpected juxtapositions and, finally, create space for fugitive thoughts and feelings through reverie, memory and desire.

Ideally, the psychotherapist reaches that space of fertile ground to make her own poetry with patients. She reflects on her use of language and tone. She threads disparate ideas together to get a fresh slant. She holds the patient with her words while he faces painful truths. Using her judgment, she is willing to reveal herself and most importantly, link her imagination with that of the patient. If she finds a poem on point, she might read it to her patient or even read it together. Together the dyad finds poetic "truth."

The clinician should also not be afraid to use strange words in strange combinations. The patient may enjoy the surprise and struggle to understand. Remember what Clarice Lispector (2012, p. 76) wrote in her novel Agua Viva, "And when I think a word is strange that's where it achieves the meaning." Part of *Wonderland*'s appeal is Carroll's unusual use of language. As W.H. Auden (1971, p. 9) writes, "... one of the most important and powerful characters [in the Alice books] is not a person but the English language." Carroll draws the reader into his magic as he unlocks words from their context and gives them an identity of their own. Carroll viewed language as living and organic, and clinicians can as well.

Who is not astonished when hearing the beginning of Carroll's poem "The Jabberwocky"?

> 'Twas brillig, and the slithy toves
> Did gyre and gimble in the wabe:
> All mimsy were the borogoves,
> And the mome raths outgrabe.'
>
> (Carroll, 2000, p. 215)

In this poem Carroll startles his reader and encourages imaginative involvement. The "lack of sense" takes us into unconscious territory, allowing the reader to associate and infer his own meaning, yet there is also a suggestion of meaning – as some words are combinations of real words. Just as we understand a patient from his nonverbal communication, we understand Jabberwocky from its tone, half-meanings and rhythms. The pattern of sounds in this first stanza of the poem imply that this is the start of a story and the stage is being set. The poem goes on to tell a familiar narrative, of a young hero who goes out to slay a monster (the Jabberwock) and, after tests of his bravery, is victorious. Carroll repeats this same first stanza at the end, suggesting the hero returns home. Because the narrative is familiar, Carroll can take even more risks with strange sounds. Similarly, our patients' narratives are familiar to them, so all the more reason to use strange sounds to help them grasp their story in a new way. The poem demonstrates what linguists call productivity or open-endedness, meaning the users of a language can endlessly compose new words or phrases. Clinicians want patients to realize they can create new sounds, phrases and perspectives for themselves. As they do so, eventually the non-sense of the unconscious will make sense.

Forgetting and remembering

The trauma victim lives "in emptiness ... gone from the minds of others" (Zornberg, referring to the biblical Joseph, 1995, p. 292). Yet, this absent state can be a starting point; the loss contains the seeds of recovery. The patient must first become aware of, that is, "remember" this absence, which the therapist helps the patient identify. A genuine awareness of loss is the only hope for recovery.

The biblical Joseph[6] experiences severe trauma. Of Jacob's 12 sons, he is the favorite, creating intense jealousy among his many half-brothers. Joseph also unwittingly goads his brothers by telling them how he sees them bow down to him in his dreams. Enraged, the brothers strip him and throw him into a pit (a void) but then decide to sell him into slavery to passing traders en route to Egypt. The brothers tell Jacob that his son Joseph is dead.

In Egypt Joseph is placed in the home of Potiphar, captain of the Pharaoh's guard. Potiphar's wife tries to seduce Joseph; after he refuses, she accuses him of rape. He is imprisoned, thrown into a second void. Due to his ability to interpret dreams, he earns the favor of the Pharaoh and is released. Eventually Joseph is appointed viceroy of Egypt, second in command to Pharaoh. He is married into Egyptian royalty and has two sons named Manasseh and Ephriam. Zornberg (1995) describes how Joseph struggles to forget his trauma yet eventually tries to piece together parts of his broken identity.[7]

During the famine that Joseph himself predicted when he analyzed Pharaoh's dreams,[8] his half-brothers come to Egypt seeking grain. Unbeknownst to them, they meet with Joseph who then remembers their abuse. At first, he is vengefully angry and falsely accuses them of stealing and spying. Finally, the brothers fully "remember" what they have done and express guilt and remorse. Touched deeply, Joseph becomes more aware of his loss. Weeping intensely, he identifies himself. Both to alleviate his brothers' guilt and to console himself, Joseph reframes their cruelty. He states it was God's will that eventually brought good. To some extent, the family reconciles, and Joseph forgives.

The Joseph story contains many of the themes therapists see in their work with trauma patients: the struggle to both remember and forget; the intense rage; the search for a healing narrative; the difficulty in reframing memories; and the question of forgiveness.

While the patient must become aware of the trauma, he cannot be overwhelmed. Entering transitional apace, working with dreams, being companionable with the patient, understanding unconscious communication, recognizing dysfunctional patterns and encouraging creative expression all help the patient process and work through his trauma. The clinician's use of language can give the patient courage to experiment and perhaps reframe his memories. I encourage the poet in all of you to take risks. However, here we heed the alchemists and their dictum, "Hurry slowly," meaning we have to be careful with the heat. Direct fire scorches and burns. We strive to find balance to help the patient land in the space of imagination.

As discussed, creative expression can allow the victim to safely reexperience trauma as it provides a witness to suffering, an antidote to aloneness. It can be a responsive, soothing presence, helping the patient step outside the trauma yet dive in and reexperience it at the same time. The aesthetic imagination can facilitate working through shock and terror in a secure place.

In the biblical narrative, Jacob went into intense grief when he was told Joseph was dead. Then years later, after the brothers reunite with Joseph, they are worried about the shock to their father if they tell him Joseph is alive. Based in Midrashic tradition, Thomas Mann (2005) develops the narrative that the brothers arrange for a young poet and musician to sing to Jacob, inviting him to remember his trauma as well as his longing and hope. Moved by the beauty of her song, Jacob is lulled into a dream-like state. When the brothers come and tell him the truth, he is more open and able to absorb what they tell him. This is an example of the power of art to help the person become more receptive and comprehend the "truth."

The adaptive imagination

Individually, we are creative at our biological core, on a cellular level. This allows us to encounter problematic situations with flexibility. Many times, our bodies respond spontaneously to assaults and devise an adaptation or compensation. The body can also learn. The immune system can be taught to remain on after it would normally turn off, so it can combat cancer. Once the body learns to fight the cancer, it will *remember* and be able to do so after the treatment ends. This parallels the psychological adaption that occurs in psychotherapy. The patient's brain changes as he or she learns to fight dysfunctional patterns and develop new possibilities. When psychotherapy is successful, new long-term memories form, and we continue to evolve, even after the treatment has ended.

In the grand sweep of evolution, we see aspects of a creative process at work. Evolution has generated the myriad unique and adaptive forms of life that have lived and died on our earth for hundreds of millions of years. Evolution can make an organism only 3 mm long that is capable of flying, has vision, sustains itself by converting chemicals into energy and is even able to reproduce (a fly) – while human technology cannot yet do that. Many times, the technology of the natural world is vastly superior to our human technology.

Solutions have existed in nature long before humans were able to "discover" them: pumps and valves in our heart, heat exchange systems used by termites to ventilate their mounds, optical lenses in our eyes and sonar used by bats, dolphins and whales (French, 1994). Bentley and Corne (2002) cite how many of our recent designs borrow features directly from evolutionary forces, such as the cross-sectional shape of aircraft wings from birds and Velcro from certain types of sticky seeds. The inventors of these products were visionaries who could use the genius of evolution to create products for our use.

Using adaptive imagination, Bentley (1999) and Bentley and Corne (2002) describe how the principles of natural evolution can be applied to computers, giving them the ability to generate creative solutions. Through a process called evolutionary design, the computer is programmed to evolve designs and produce creative products in many fields, including visual arts, music, product design and architecture, harnessing the power of evolution for non-living designs. This is an emergent process and not explicitly stated in the algorithm (Bentley, 1999), frequently surprising the researchers who write them. The researchers cannot predict the outcome of a program until it is runs (Lehman et al., 2018), just as our patients can surprise us and develop in ways not previously imagined.

It is necessary to understand the gene to understand evolution (Mukherjee, 2016). For evolution to occur, both variation and stability are necessary. The gene must mutate, that is, change its DNA sequence and produce variations. The gene, in fact, is malleable. The rate of mutation or variation is surprising, which is positive. Without the possibility of deep genetic diversity, an organism could lose the ability to survive in changing circumstances.

Variation is also crucial for psychological imagination. To advance our field, we cannot just repeat what is already known. We need twists and turns to discover new approaches, which we integrate with our stable body of knowledge. Interdisciplinary exploration is a help in this regard.

In our work with patients, we ask: is the therapy "hurrying slowly" with a good blend of empathy and confrontation? Have there been some "aha" moments to provide variation and catalyze the process? Therapy usually proceeds at a relatively slow pace but must also welcome sudden change.

Endings

All creation contains some sadness, as the work eventually separates from the creator: the child from the parent, the patient from the therapist, this volume from me. Reader and writer (you and I) also terminate, as poignant for us as it can be for patient and therapist.

I understand the pain and confusion of separation. To be transparent, I am obsessed with reuniting with people who have died long ago. For years I fantasized about my dead relatives coming alive, just for an hour or two, so I could talk to them, ask them questions and maybe find some answers. I have often bargained with God just to have one more hour with each of them. This led me to write a semiautobiographical play, *The Meeting of My Dreams*,[9] in which five generations of matriarchs (three of whom are dead) meet and, through the analysis of dreams, begin to understand each other and, in some cases, forgive.

In psychotherapy, therapist and patient swim in uncertainty and live with paradox and mystery. The therapist listens carefully to her patient, many times feeling puzzled, not really understanding the unconscious communication. Then suddenly she may become aware of an important underlying dynamic and can offer a clarification or interpretation that makes sense of the chaos. Slowly, over time, clinicians grow to savor the mysteries of psychotherapy and, when it occurs, the ensuing feeling of clarity. The leap out of chaos is addictive, in the best sense of the word.

Psychotherapy is a creative process. We are confused, we get glimmers of insight, we lose that, we reflect, we are aware of many opposing forces in our patient and ourselves, we lower our boundaries, we give up our habitual ideas, we sit with our patient until an insight gels and then finally, we can bring something to the patient that moves him. We want the patient to be comfortable in his confusion *and* in his clarity – and the same for you, dear Reader. As we part, my wish for you is to dwell in wonder, listen for surprise, catch hold of the uncanny, "dance" with the patient, and, most importantly, continue to dream for yourself and your patient.

Notes

1 *Havdalah* is a Jewish religious ceremony that marks the end of the sacred time of the Sabbath and the beginning of the rest of the days of the week.
2 *Temenos* is a Greek word for sanctuary or sacred and protected space. Jung applied this concept to the protected and protective space of the therapeutic relationship. https://www.psychceu.com/Juand protectedng/sharplexicon.html
3 Cummings, E.E. (1994). I thank You God for most this amazing. In R.S. Kennedy (Ed.), *Selected Poems* (p. 167). New York: Norton.
4 Williams, W.C. (1991). The Red Wheelbarrow. In A.W. Litz & C. MacGowan (Eds.), *The collected poems of William Carlos Williams: Volume 1: 1909–1939* (p. 224). New York: New Directions.
5 Stevens, W. (2015). Notes Towards a Supreme Fiction, In C. Beyers & J. Serio (Eds.), *The collected poems: The corrected edition* (p. 401). New York: Vintage Books.

6 Although the culture and customs of the time period of Genesis, approximately 3,500 years ago, are very different from current times, I am reading the story of Joseph and his brothers as literature. The uncanny universality of the themes is relevant today.
7 Joseph names his two sons, Manasseh and Efraim, after the motif of forgetting and remembering. Manasseh means forgetfulness. According to the Torah commentary of Naftali Zvi Yehuda Berlin, known as the Netziv, in choosing this name, Joseph recognizes the blessing of being able to forget the loss of his family and spiritual heritage (Zornberg, 1995). He has to survive, and painful yearnings for his past would distract him. This is a form of adaptive dissociation. Ephriam means fruitful. Able to be lifegiving even in this land of suffering, Joseph not only becomes the father of two sons but, as viceroy of Egypt, also the preserver and distributer of food to many nations during the famine (Zornberg, 1995). In these acts, he is weaving his narrative of trauma, resilience and reconstitution, examples of the "art of trauma."
8 Joseph anticipated the famine when he was called to interpret Pharaoh's dreams: first, seven sick, lean cows eating seven plump cows and second, seven thin ears of grain eating seven plump ears. Joseph foretold that Egypt would experience seven years of plenty followed by seven years of severe famine and advised Pharaoh to store grain. Pharaoh then appointed Joseph as viceroy in charge of preparing for the famine.
9 *The Meeting of My Dreams*, a theatrical presentation, had the following performances: April 26, 2015, 35th Annual Spring Meeting of the Division of Psychoanalysis (39) of the American Psychological Association, *Life in Psychoanalysis in Life*; July 19, 2015, Society for Exploration of Psychoanalytic Therapies and Theology, Allentown, PA.

References

Auden, W.H. (1971). Today's 'wonder-world' needs Alice. In R. Phillips (Ed.), *Aspects of Alice: Lewis Carroll's dreamchild as seen through the critics' looking-glasses, 1865–1971* (pp. 3–12). New York: Vanguard.

Bentley, P.J. (1999). Is evolution creative? In P.J. Bentley & D.W. Corne (Eds.), *Proceedings of the AISB'99 symposium on creative evolutionary systems (CES)*. Published by The Society for the Study of Artificial Intelligence and Stimulation of Behaviour (AISB), (pp. 28–34).

Bentley, P.J. & Corne, D.W. (2002). An introduction to creative evolutionary systems. In P.J. Bentley and D.W. Corne (Eds.), *Creative evolutionary systems* (pp. 1–75). San Diego, CA: Academic Press.

Bion, W.R. (1962). *Learning from experience*. London: Heinemann.

Bollas, C. (1979). The transformational object. *International Journal of Psycho-Analysis*, 60:97–107.

Bollas, C. (2017). *The shadow of the object: Psychoanalysis of the unthought known*. New York: Columbia University Press.

Bromberg, P.M. (2000). Bringing in the dreamer: Some reflections on dreamwork, surprise, and the analytic process. *Contemporary Psychoanalysis*, 36:685–705.

Carroll, L. (2000). J. Gardner (Introduction and notes), *The annotated Alice: The definitive edition*. Original illustrations by J. Tenniel. New York: Norton.

Csikszentmihalyi, M. (1996). *Creativity: Flow and the psychology of discovery and invention*. New York: Harper Collins.

Darwin, C. (1879/2004). *The descent of man*. New York: Penguin.
Domash, L. (2009). The emergence of hope: Implicit spirituality in treatment and the occurrence of psychoanalytic luck. *Psychoanalytic Review*, 96:35–54.
Domash, L. (2010). Unconscious freedom and the insight of the analyst: Exploring neuropsychological processes underlying 'aha' moments. *Journal of The American Academy of Psychoanalysis and Dynamic Psychiatry*, 38:315–339.
French, M.J. (1994). *Invention and Evolution: Design in Nature and Engineering*, Second edition. Cambridge, UK: Cambridge University Press.
Knoblauch, S.H. (2005). Body rhythms and the unconscious: Toward an expanding of clinical attention. *Psychoanalytic Dialogues*, 15(6):807–827.
Lehman, J., Clune, J., Misevic, D., Adami, C., Altenberg, L., Beaulieu, J., Bentley, P.J. Bernard, S., Beslon, G., Bryson, D.M., Chrabaszcz, P., Cheney, N., Cully, A., Doncieux, S., Dyer, F.C., Ellefsen, K.O., Feldt, R., Fischer, S., Forrest, S., Frénoy, A., Gagné, C., LeGoff, L., Grabowski, L.M., Hodjat, B., Hutter, F., et al. (28 additional authors not shown). (2018). The surprising creativity of digital evolution: A collection of anecdotes from the evolutionary computation and artificial life research communities. arXiv Labs, Cornell University. arXiv:1803.03453v3 [cs.NE]
Lispector, C. (2012). *Agua viva*. New York: New Directions.
Mann, T. (2005). *Joseph and his brothers: The stories of Jacob, young Joseph, Joseph in Egypt, Joseph the provider*. New York: Knopf.
Marks-Tarlow, T. (2012). *Clinical intuition in psychotherapy: The neurobiology of embodied response*. New York: Norton.
Mukherjee, S. (2016). *The gene: An intimate history*. New York: Scribner.
Poland, W. (1975). Tact as a psychoanalytic function. *International Journal of Psycho-Analysis*, 56:155–162.
Reik, T. (1936). *Surprise and the psycho-analyst*. London: Kegan Paul, Trench, Tru & Co.
Starr, K. (2008). *Repair of the soul: Metaphors of transformation in Jewish mysticism and psychoanalysis*. New York: Routledge.
Steiner, G. (1989). *Real presences*. Chicago, IL: University of Chicago Press.
Stern, D.B. (1990). Courting surprise – Unbidden perceptions in clinical practice. *Contemporary Psychoanalysis*, 26:452–478.
Zelnick, L. (2014). Narrative surprise: Relational psychoanalytic process and biblical text. *DIVISION/Review*, 9:33.
Zornberg, A. (1995). *The beginnings of desire: Reflections on Genesis*. New York: Schocken Books.

Index

Note: Page numbers followed by "n" denote endnotes.

For Product Safety Concerns and Information please contact our EU representative GPSR@taylorandfrancis.com
Taylor & Francis Verlag GmbH, Kaufingerstraße 24, 80331 München, Germany

www.ingramcontent.com/pod-product-compliance
Ingram Content Group UK Ltd.
Pitfield, Milton Keynes, MK11 3LW, UK
UKHW020203200926
475702UK00004B/589

* 9 7 8 0 3 6 7 2 8 0 0 2 4 *